IMMUNOGENETICS AND DISEASES

Dr. Kavita Ramanathan

ALLIED HEALTH PRESS

Immunogenetics and Diseases

Author: **Dr. Kavita Ramanathan**

Allied Health Press
4164 Lakeshore Road
Burlington ON L7L 1A4
Canada
www.alliedhealthpress.com
Email: orders@arclereducation.com

ISBN: 978-1-77956-766-6

Allied Health Press publishes wide variety of books and eBooks. For more information about Allied Health Press and its products, visit our website at www.alliedhealthpress.com

ABOUT THE AUTHOR

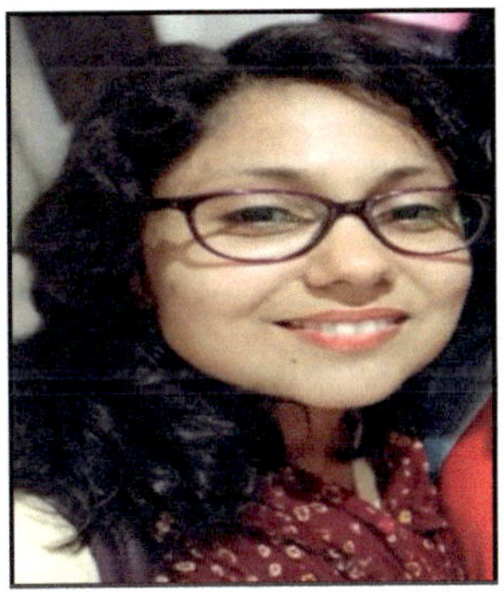

Dr Kavita Ramanathan is an accomplished medical professional with experience working through the length and breadth of India. With 16+ years in clinical and anatomic pathology, she understands the normal and abnormal functioning of the human body in depth. Also, she held positions in the senior management for 8+ years and designed business strategies. She successfully helped organisations attain profitability while maintaining quality and service standards. Additionally, during the COVID-19 pandemic, she contributed significantly by aligning operations to support government initiatives. She earned her undergraduate and graduate medical degrees from reputed institutions under the University of Mumbai, India, and she also holds an MBA in Finance. Dr Kavita volunteers with a non-profit organisation where she tutors students from low-income schools for over two decades. Post-pandemic, she quit her corporate job to pursue her passion of teaching and writing. Currently, she tutors high school and university students in biology, psychology, and medical sciences. Additionally, she authors books, articles, and blogs on topics related to health and well-being. Her strong academic background, enriched with a vast and varied experience, shapes her into a mature and sensible professional.

Brief Table of Contents

Detailed Table of Contents

LIST OF FIGURES

PREFACE

The immune system has complex mechanism, many of which are under study. Loss of self-tolerance, cellular infiltration into the target organs, and local inflammation are all examples of the coordinated sequence of events that culminate in autoimmune disease. Growth factors, cytokines, antibodies, adhesion molecules, and other chemicals cause and control vital cell processes that sustain inflammation, resulting in tissue damage and symptoms. The distinct amino acid sequences that characterize allelic variants on each of the many molecules influence the type and severity of this reaction as well as the capacity to return to homeostasis. Genes are largely responsible for defining the risk of developing such disorders, the course of the condition, and how well the patients respond to treatment. Despite the obvious presence of genetic factors in many disorders, progress has been delayed by the inability to fully utilize traditional genetic epidemiologic tools due to the absence of consistent means of transmission. Moreover, autoimmune disorders are distinguished by complex interactions with environmental factors and moderate heredity of disease risk. However, many recent findings have altered our capacity to investigate genetic variation in relation to human disease. There has been advancement in the use of novel analytical and data-management techniques in recent years, in addition to the production of extensive laboratory techniques for effectively identifying and cataloging DNA diversity. Advancements in data mining are enabling the analysis of genetic networks sustaining biological processes as well as the identification of co-regulated genes. These developments, along with the rising costs of autoimmune disorders to society, offer a compelling reason to investigate how genetics and genomes contribute to the pathogenic disruption of immunological homeostasis. Gaining insight into the genetic causes of these conditions may help identify the fundamental causes of the disease, which will result in improved treatment options as well as potential preventative measures.

Fungal infections are thought to affect more than a billion people annually, and new data indicates that the number is rising. There are no vaccines, and treating invasive fungal infections (IFDs) is a difficult task with intolerable mortality and morbidity rates, especially in immunocompromised hosts and critically ill patients. Hematologic diseases, solid organ or stem cell transplantation, primary or acquired immunodeficiencies, immunosuppressive therapy, and prolonged intensive care unit treatment are critical risk factors for IFD. Even though a wide range of antifungal medications or drugs are available, the evaluation of host-derived indicators of susceptibility and diagnostic techniques that do not enable an accurate diagnosis of infection frequently provide obstacles to the effective treatment of IFD. Even among individuals with comparable underlying clinical conditions and microbiological exposure, there are differences in the likelihood of IFD. Susceptibility to IA is believed to primarily depend on genetic predisposition. The DNA sequences in each individual cells are nearly identical. This suggests that genetic information alone is insufficient to explain the variations in gene expression that occur throughout cell differentiation and development. Over the past years, research has also demonstrated the significance of a variety of complex epigenetic processes, including DNA cytosine methylation, covalent modifications of histones, and specific forms of RNA interference, that control transcription by altering chromatin conformation. Several residues in histones can be altered by different processes, including phosphorylation, acetylation, methylation, and ubiquitination.

INTRODUCTION

The routine diagnostic immunogenetics laboratory has to characterize the HLA and other genes within the MHC to assist solid organ and hemopoietic stem cell transplant programs. HLA typing by molecular methods, such as direct DNA sequencing, sequence-specific oligonucleotide hybridization (SSO) and sequence-specific priming (SSP) techniques, and the use of specialized software for HLA allele assignment, are important. There are several molecular techniques designed for the typing of particular HLA alleles that are useful for diagnosing diseases and hypersensitivity reactions. The HLA molecules HLA-E and HLA-G, the MICA genes, and single nucleotide polymorphisms (SNPs) across the MHC are among the MHC genes that are important. The type of healthcare that has been envisioned since the early 20th century with the introduction of disease-based medicine will be made possible by genome-based data. Physicians will be able to fulfill their goal of providing the individualized medical care possible if a system of healthcare is developed that leverages the data intensity of the genome and its derivatives in addition to imaging, clinical, and environmental data. However, as healthcareconsumers, this information will also enable each of us to adopt a more proactive attitude to health. We are at the beginning of a significant shift in our knowledge of the biological foundations of health and disease as well as in the prediction capacity of science and medicine. The immune system communicates with different cell types inside or outside the immune system through soluble chemicals called cytokines, which are produced by immune cells. At every stage of the development of autoimmune disease, including the production of pathogenic or protective effector cells, the trafficking of pathogenic cells to the target organ, and the mediation of tissue damage or tissue tolerance in the target organ, cytokines form a network of soluble effector molecules. Naive autoreactive T cells undergo differentiation into cells that generate proinflammatory or anti-inflammatory cytokines after being activated. Autoreactive cells that produce anti-inflammatory cytokines may, but do not always, prevent autoimmune disorders, while pathogenic cells that produce proinflammatory cytokines cause organ-specific autoimmune diseases. Autoimmune diseases may be prevented or reversed by interventions aimed at reducing the production of proinflammatory cytokines or the differentiation of cells into proinflammatory phenotypes, or, increasing anti-inflammatory cytokines or the differentiation of cells into anti-inflammatory phenotypes. This demonstrates how cytokine regulation has a therapeutic potential for the management of autoimmune disorders.

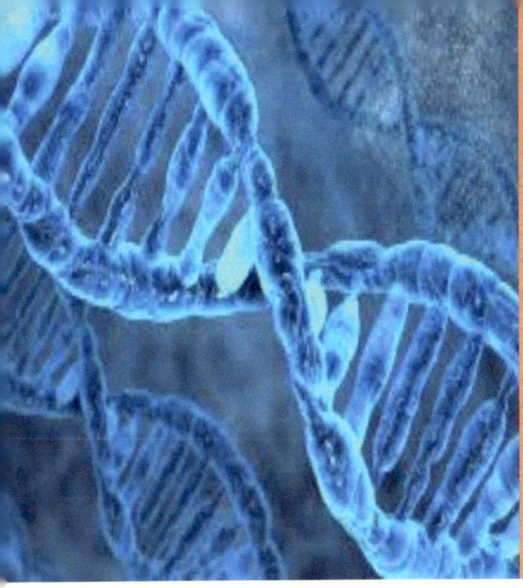

Chapter 1

INTRODUCTION TO IMMUNOGENETICS

Contents

1.1 Introduction

Immunogenetics is the study of a set of biological processes that are involved in the immune system and controlled by its genes(Rashid et al., 2022). A genetic condition that affects immune system development makes a person more prone to autoimmunity and cancer as well as unable to prevent infections. Immunology is the science that studies how the body fights infections and how such defenses can malfunction. As molecular genetics has advanced, so too has our understanding of the genetic and molecular basis of immune response. The immune system is made up of two parts, both of which come from the same precursor stem cells. When appropriately activated, B lymphocytes produce plasma cells.

These plasma cells develop into immunoglobulins or antibodies. Usually, antigens cause the production of antibodies. These antibodies trigger humoral immunity, in which they identify the antigen and eliminate it. Another subclass of cells known as T cells mediates all of these interactions. An improved immune response occurs when B cells contact a specific antigen because they recognize it for use in subsequent attacks. This is known as immunological memory. Understanding the genetic regulation of immunoglobulin synthesis is the primary challenge in comprehending the genetic foundation of immune response(Rabinovich et al., 2012). A single gene can produce a large number of antibodies, or different genes can produce different classes of antibodies. Recombinant technology has provided answers to these questions by demonstrating how a small number of genes may encode a large number of antibodies. The heavy and lighter chains are two of the many distinct polypeptide chains that make up each antibody. The protein components of the two chains differ. In antibodies, these chains contain both constant and variable regions. The specificity of each antibody is determined by the various amino acid sequences in the variable sections compared to the identical amino acid sequence in the constant regions.

1.2 Blood type

Mendelian inheritance of human blood types was demonstrated in 1910, which is when immunogenetics first emerged. Antibodies were used to identify a large number of blood groups. The discovery of goat blood groups by P. Ehrlich and J. Morgen Roth in the early 20th century marked the beginning of the field of immunogenetics(Irwin, 1976).

Karl Landsteiner identified the human blood groups known as ABO blood types in 1901(Wiener, 1966) (Figure 1). He began his lab experiment by drawing blood samples from each of his colleagues and separating the plasma from the cellular components. The findings following sample mixing were quite interesting; he found that RBC clumped together when combined with sera from various people, and that same agglutination also occurred when human and animal blood were combined. These findings demonstrated the existence of blood group variation. Based on this experiment, the human blood groups were designated as A and B. Group A blood agglutinates with group B, but never with its own type, according to Landsteiner. Group C blood is unique in that it agglutinates with both A and B, while group B blood agglutinates with group A. Red blood cells stick/clump together to form agglutinin because their surface contains antigens that react with plasma antibodies, which are a crucial component of the immunological response. The concept of agglutinin, or antibodies, which provide the basis of the antibody-antigen response in the ABO complex, was presented along with this particular blood group interaction, which was named isoagglutination.

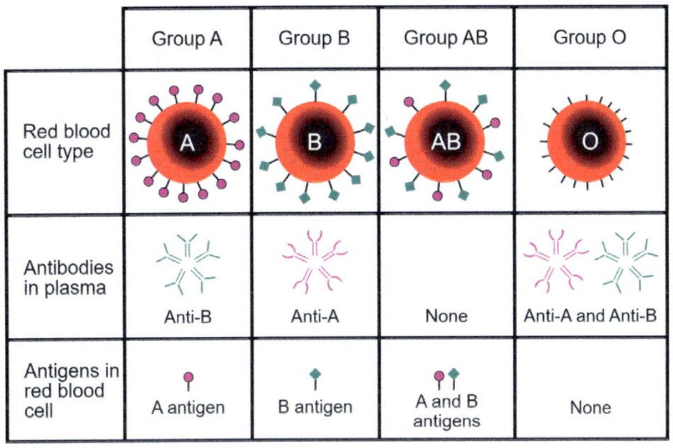

Figure 1.1 ABO blood types

Source: https://commons.wikimedia.org/wiki/File:ABO_blood_type.svg,*Creative Commons License.*

These blood groups have developed in humans, and a person's blood group is always determined by the distinct gene set they inherit from their parents. Immunogenetics includes more than just the study of blood types and how they interact. The field of immunogenetics began in 1976 when Edward Jenner discovered that cowpox might be used to prevent smallpox since those who had previously had cowpox were immune to smallpox. All of the blood-type antigens found on the outside of red blood cells have been shown to be completely distinct from one another. The information contained in genes controls the properties of various antigens. As a result, both individual and cell peculiarities are genetically determined. When cells with different external characteristics come into contact with one another, a reaction occurs in the individual that can lead to tissue transplantation. Pregnant women are an exception, as their father's genes have fixed antigens on the membranes of the fetal cells. Consequently, the immune system's reaction to foreign transplants is crucial for ensuring that cells maintain their unique surface characteristics, even though these characteristics may alter in the event of a viral infection or when a healthy cell transforms into a malignant one. The tendency to distinguish between self and nonself is extremely important. Maintaining a healthy defense system is crucial; otherwise, autoimmune diseases would increase. It has been discovered that an individual's genetic composition regulates their immune response to a foreign entity. Each person experiences protection mechanisms in a different way. It indicates that the response is inherited.

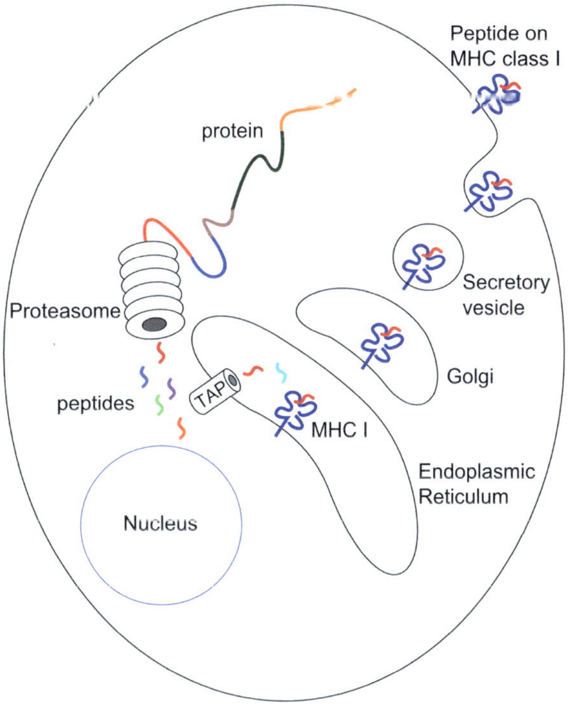

Figure 1.2 Major Histocompatibilty Complex (MHC)

Source: https://upload.wikimedia.org/wikipedia/commons/d/d7/MHC_Class_I_processing.svg,*Creative Commons License.*

1.3 Major Histocompatibilty Complex

The majority of vertebrates contain the Major Histocompatibilty Complex (MHC) gene family

(Figure 1.2). The MHC has more than 200 coding loci and a significant amount of DNA that spans over 4 million base pairs in humans, or 0.1% of the human genome(Geraghty et al., 2002). The MHC cluster is found on chromosome 17 in mice (Figure 3).

Human chromosome 6 contains a locus with three subfamilies (grouped or clustered); class III is found between MHC classes I and II (Figure 4). MHC class I and II genes are highly polymorphic loci found in vertebrates that influence immunological self/nonself reactions. All nucleated somatic cells have class I glycoproteins on their surface, but MHC class II glycoproteins are found in specialized antigen-presenting cells (APCs), including B cells, dendritic cells, and macrophages. Peptides (antigens) that are intrinsic to CD^{8+} cytotoxic T cells (CTLs) are presented by MHC class I molecules. Regarding MHC class II, they present antigens that are external to CD^{4+} helper T (TH) cells. Through antigen presentation, MHC regulates distinct immune responses mediated by both cells and antibodies(Jiang & Chess, 2000).

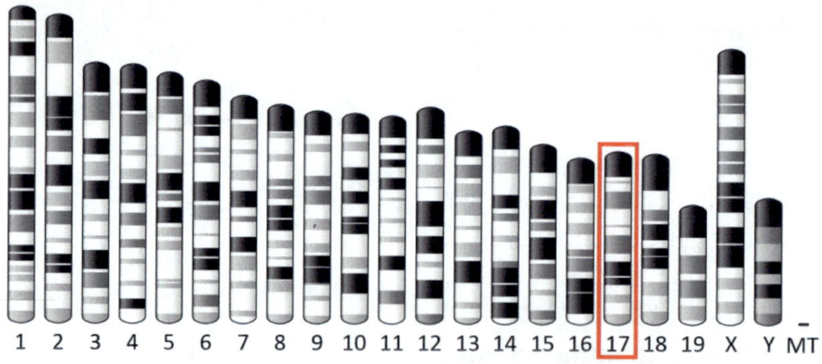

Figure 1.3 Chromosome 17 in mice

Source: https://upload.wikimedia.org/wikipedia/commons/1/13/Ideogram_house_mouse_chromosome_17.svg,*Creative Commons License.*

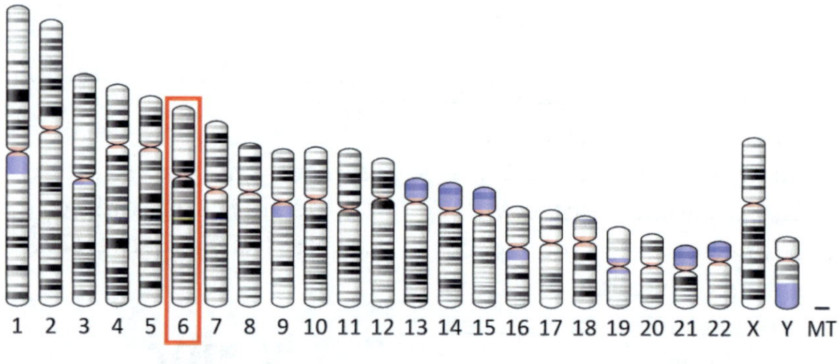

Figure 1.4 Chromosome 6 in humans

Source: https://upload.wikimedia.org/wikipedia/commons/0/03/Ideogram_human_chromosome_6.svg,*Creative Commons License.*

MHC genes are researched to know the genetic systems because they regulate important characteristics like resistance to infectious diseases. MHC was identified because of its interesting role in tissue transplantation. It nearly took 20 years after MHC discovery to comprehend its biological function in peptide presentation and T-cell response. T cell primary functions include defending the body from invasion and triggering B lymphocytes and macrophages. T cells must interact with other cells, including B lymphocytes, dendritic cells, macrophages, and infected host cells, to activate. B cell receptors can identify antigens on the cell surface, whereas T cells can identify antigens on other cells. Protein molecules that are expressed by genes in a region known as MHC display these cellular antigens. Depending on how well the two genetic loci match, the genes in these loci determine the outcome of the tissue donation. The primary characteristic of MHC loci is their polymorphism, which results in different gene forms.

1.4 Dynamics of the Major Histocompatibilty Complex (MHC)

MHC class I expresses glycoproteins known as MHC molecules on all nucleated cells. The 43 kDa transmembrane glycoprotein known as alpha or heavy chain is encoded by each MHC class I(Hassan & Ahmad, 2011). In this context, α 1, α 2, and α 3 are the three extracellular domains that make up each heavy chain. The highly conserved alpha 3 molecule interacts with the CD^8 molecule found on cytotoxic T lymphocytes. All nucleated cells exhibit class I expression, but at varying levels; lymphocytes exhibit the highest amount, whereas hepatocytes exhibit the lowest. Similar to MHC class I, class II MHC is made up of transmembrane glycoprotein molecules known as alpha 1 and 2, beta 1, and beta 2 that have extracellular domains and a cytoplasmic tail. α- and β-chains with molecular weights of roughly 35,000 and 28,000 Da, respectively, are encoded by class II MHC genes. The Ig superfamily also includes MHC class II molecules. Only APCs such as B lymphocytes, dendritic cells, and macrophages express molecules that are expressed by class II MHC genes. TH cells are prepared to bind and aid in antigen recognition when MHC class II molecules align antigens to the outside of the cell membrane. This class comprises all the genes linked to inflammatory factors and complement system components. This gene class codes for many proteins in the immunological response. T-cell receptors mediate the presentation of antigens. Only when the antigen is coupled with MHC molecules do these T cells identify it. MHC molecules are necessary for the presentation of antigen by both cytotoxic and helper T lymphocytes. CD^8 T cells receive the processed endogenous antigen from class I, whereas CD^4 T cells receive it from class II(Frandji et al., 1996). Endogenous antigens function in distinct ways. Most of the autoimmune diseases impact between 3 and 10% of the global population. It was discovered that autoimmune diseases and genetic factors were closely related. Certain alleles of the HLA-Dr and HL-ADQ genes have been linked to a tendency to a number of these autoimmune disorders. Through the retrieval of pattern recognition receptors (PRRs), such as Toll-like receptors (TLRs), and signal transducing particles, such as interleukin-1 receptor associated kinase 4 (IRAK4), the innate immune system establishes the primary defense against foreign antigens.

1.5 Autoimmune diseases

The abnormal activity (low) results in a lack of recognition of external influences (factors), which actually predisposes the person to infection. The body will be more vulnerable to autoimmune and infectious diseases if something is obstructing the immune system activity. Immunogenetics focuses on the effects of both HLA and non-HLA on autoimmune disorders and infections. Rheumatoid arthritis (RA) is a painful inflammatory condition that affects joints, including the hands and feet. The immune system of the patient tends to target its own tissues in this disease. In extreme situations, the internal organs are also impacted. About 5-7 million Indians are afflicted with the disease, and the number of cases has risen to 1 million annually in India alone(Gupta, 2004). Although there is no cure for this disease, medical intervention can help it grow more slowly. The development of autoantibodies against post-translationally changed proteins is the first step in the long-term immunopathogenesis of rheumatoid arthritis. Following this gradual immune system remodeling, tissue tolerance deteriorates and becomes inflamed as a result of effector T cell production and macrophage inability to offer adequate defense. The disease changes from acute to chronic as a result of effector cells being more aggressive. It has been discovered that telomere fragility and instability of mitochondrial DNA are caused by a defect in the mitochondrial DNA repair machinery. The autoimmune disease aberrant signaling pathways are caused by cells such as macrophages, monocytes, fibroblasts, and T cells, which generate a variety of cytokines like interluekin (IL)-1, IL-6, and tumor necrosis factor (TNF)-α. MHC class II genes have been shown to be strongly associated with RA. A typical amino acid sequence found in the HLA-DBR1 region is present in this MHC locus. Certain non-HLA loci have also been linked to RA.

A chronic autoimmune skin disorder called psoriasis is characterized by aberrant keratinocyte growth(Ayala-Fontánez et al., 2016) (Figure 1.5). Psoriasis skin lesions are characterized by aberrant keratinocyte development and inflammatory cell percolation. This disease affects 2% to 3% of the population, impairing quality of life and causing long-term life impairment. This disease pathophysiology is not well understood. In more serious cases, it may put the patient at risk for a number of mental, cardiovascular, and other issues. Overactivation of T helper cells result in an excess of cytokines, including interferon gamma (IFN-γ), IL2, IL12, and tumor necrosis factor(Jorgovanovic et al., 2020). It has been observed that dendritic cell presentation of antigen to T lymphocytes contributes to the development of plaque in psoriasis patients. The risk genes for psoriasis have been identified as over 60 distinct gene loci. However, it has also been noted that approximately 50% of psoriasis patients have the MHC class I gene allele.

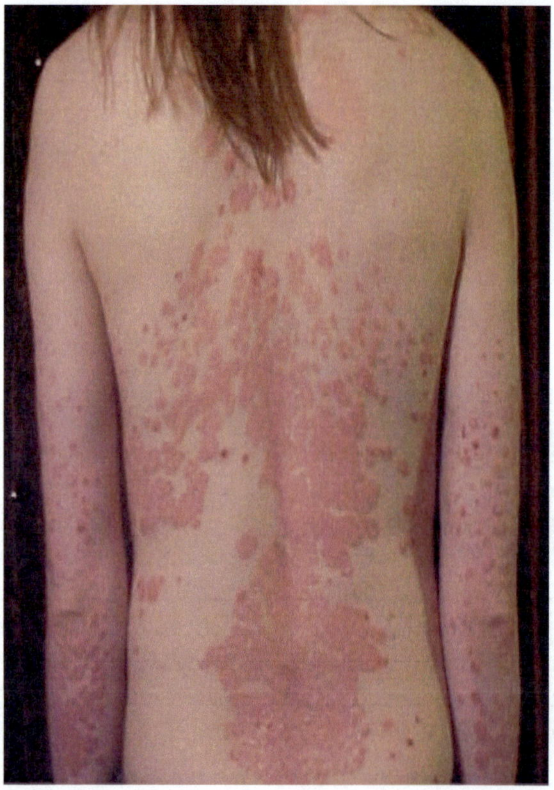

Figure 1.5 Psoriasis

Source: https://upload.wikimedia.org/wikipedia/commons/f/f5/Psoriasis_on_back1.jpg,*Creative Commons License.*

Both HLA and non-HLA gene loci are thought to be mediators of macrophage activation and antigen presentation. Reducing the threshold for innate immunity stimulation is probably a major strategy for these genetic risk alleles in the pathological phase of psoriasis. Another category of autoimmune disorders is autoimmune thyroid diseases (AITDs), which include Hashimoto's thyroiditis and Grave's disease, in which the body's own tissues are attacked by antibodies generated by the immune system. The immune system targets the thyroid gland in Hashimoto's thyroiditis (Figure 1.6), resulting in either hyperthyroidism or hypothyroidism. The fact that AITDs frequently co-occur with other autoimmune diseases makes them exceptionally significant. Although the precise method of interaction is unclear, environmental and genetic factors both play a part in this multifactorial disease. Autoimmune antibody production and thyroid gland cell infiltration identify it as a T cell-mediated disease. Further, AITDs that support T-lymphocyte activation and antigen presentation have been linked to a large number of genetic loci within HLA genes. Several cytokine Th2 gene polymorphisms have been linked to AITDs. The development of the disease is influenced by the cytokine Th2. The central and peripheral tolerance intervention, followed by T-cell activation, preserves a mechanism of immunogenetic sensitivity to AITDs.

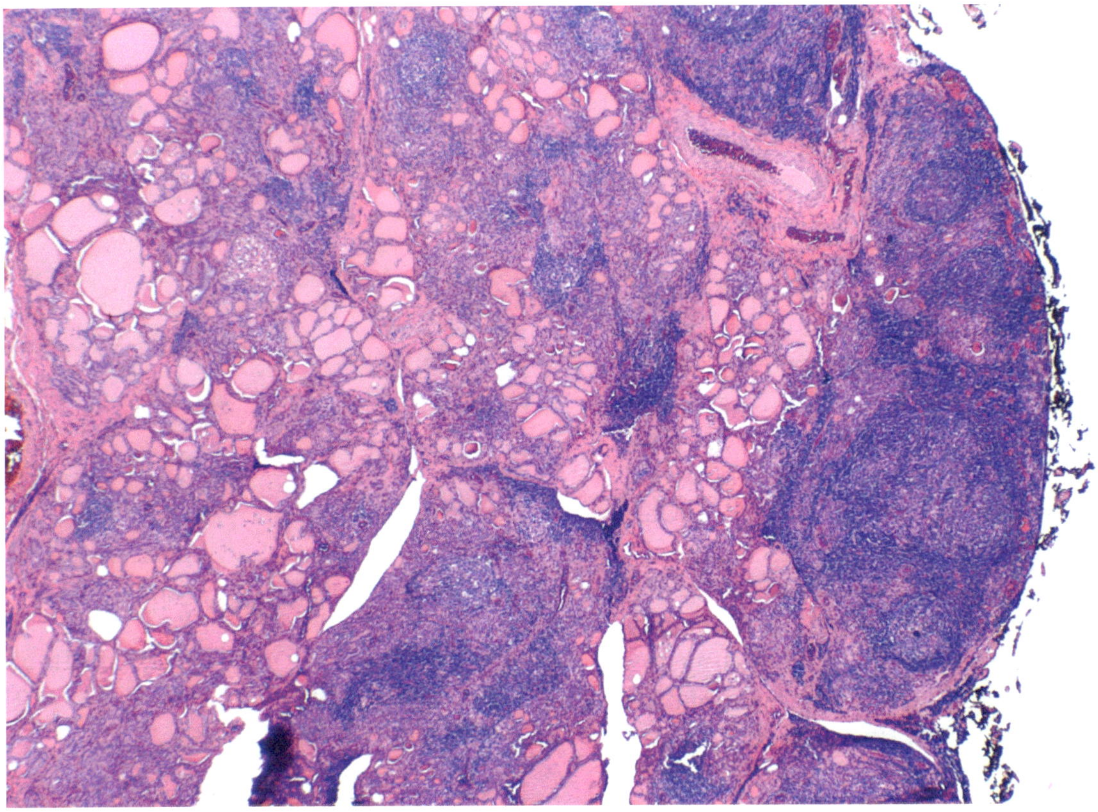

Figure 1.6 Hashimoto's thyroiditis

Source: https://upload.wikimedia.org/wikipedia/commons/5/51/Hashimoto_thyroiditis_-_alt_--_very_low_mag.jpg,*Creative Commons License.*

Primary biliary cholangitis (PBC) is a liver autoimmune disease with a hereditary component(Lleo et al., 2017). Primary biliary cirrhosis was another name for it. Women are more likely than men to have this disease. Cholestasis is a degenerative ailment that begins with the gradual blockage of the small bile ducts, which causes bile and other toxins to accumulate in the liver. Antimitochondrial antibodies (AMA) have been reported to be present in 90% of people with this disease. There is a significant rise of AMA-specific CD^{4+} and CD^{8+} T lymphocytes in the liver of PBC patients. This disease has a characteristic T cell signature. When AMA is present, macrophages exhibit enhanced expression of TNF-related apoptosis. T cell responses, such as CD^{4+} and CD^{8+} T cells, target the same antigen (Ag) and are involved in damaging biliary epithelial cells in addition to humoral response. In addition to T cells, other immune cells such as B cells, macrophages, and natural killer cells are also a part of the inflammation. The biliary epithelial cells are lost as a result of this persistent inflammation. Many genetic investigations have demonstrated that HLA variations are both protective and susceptibleto PBC. Genes linked to T cells make up the majority of non-HLA loci linked to PBC. Insulin-dependent diabetes known as type 1 diabetes mellitus (T1DM), is a complicated disease characterized by the inability to generate insulin due to the autoimmune destruction of the pancreatic beta cells. T1DM is a complex disease. Autoantibodies are produced against islet cells in type 1 diabetes, an autoimmune disease mediated by T lymphocytes(Knip & Siljander, 2008). Many susceptibility genes are involved in this genetic disease. Over half of the genetic vulnerability to type 1 diabetes is caused by polygenic HLA class II on chromosome 6 genes. Several loci that provide a protective role have also been identified. A variable number of tandem mini satellite repeats or VNTR and CTLA-4 are two HLA genes linked to type 1 diabetes (T1DM), although their effects are far less noticeable than those of HLA. Future pathophysiological insights for early intervention and disease prevention will be made possible by the discovery of new loci and further investigation of existing ones. It will assist in identifying possible sub-genotypes that exhibit distinct immune dysregulation patterns yet share disease characteristics.

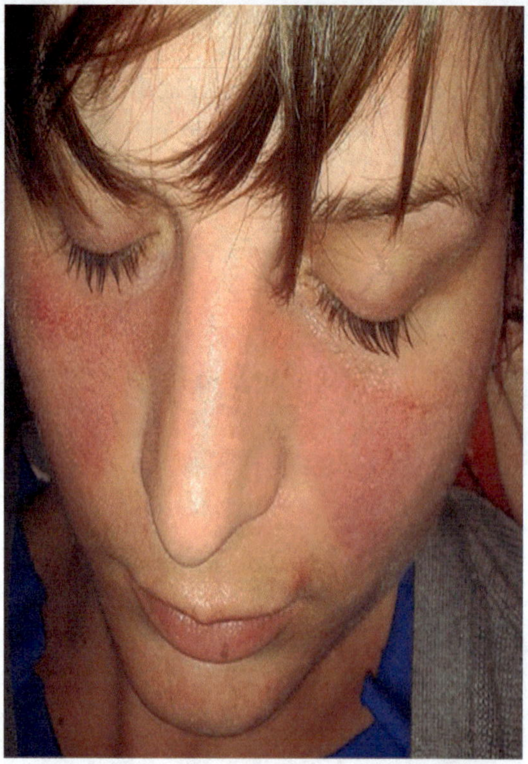

Figure 1.7 Systemic lupus erythematosus

Source: https://upload.wikimedia.org/wikipedia/commons/5/52/Lupusfoto.jpg,*Creative Commons License.*

Systemic lupus erythematosus (SLE) is an inflammatory autoimmune disease that affects several organ systems and causes organ damage (Aringer, 2020) (Figure 1.7). There are several gene loci linked to the disease vulnerability, making it a polygenic condition. A significant part of the pathophysiology of this disease is genetic. Nearly 100 loci have been linked to the disease. The pathophysiology of SLE is favored by the generation of type I interferon and autoantibodies as well as the activation of the innate immune response. Apoptosis and neutrophil extracellular traps (NET) clearance are two processes that are inhibited in SLE(Chauhan et al., 2015). The epigenetic alterations in neutrophils that ultimately result in the generation of T and B cell abnormalities are thought to be the cause of the elevated levels of cytokine generation. The NET complexes, which are elevated in SLE and have impaired clearance, are directly impacted by this epigenetic alteration in neutrophils. Both HLA and non-HLA genes are involved in this complex disease. SLE predisposition is linked to several HLA genes. They are linked to autoantibody profiles in SLE patients i.e., anti-dsDNA & anti-Ro. Nearly 100 loci have been linked to SLE by genome-wide associations. Nevertheless, it has been noted that these loci only account for around 30% of the biology of SLE in terms of effector genes and pathogenic pathways, as well as its heredity.

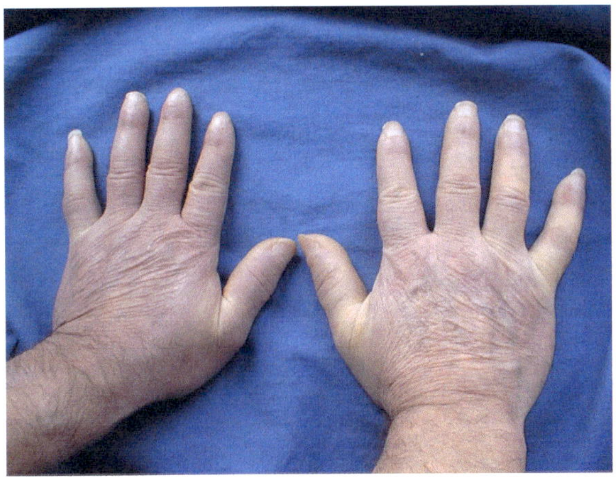

Figure 1.8 Scleroderma

Source: https://upload.wikimedia.org/wikipedia/commons/a/a3/Systemic_sclerosis%2C_changes_on_hands_are_allways_bilateral.jpg,*Creative Commons License.*

Scleroderma, (Figure 1.8) another name for systemic sclerosis (SSc), is a complicated autoimmune inflammatory disease. It is a connective tissue disease that affects the various organ systems and is characterized by vascular abnormalities that are both structural and functional. The clinical symptoms of this complex disease are diverse. Fibrosis results from an overabundance of collagen building up in the skin. MHC genes are crucial in determining a person's vulnerability to this disease. HLA-DRB1 and HPB1 are two of the several identified HLA genes that increase the risk of SSc. Regarding the non-HLA loci linked to SSc, genome scan analysis has identified approximately 28 loci as being connected to this disease.

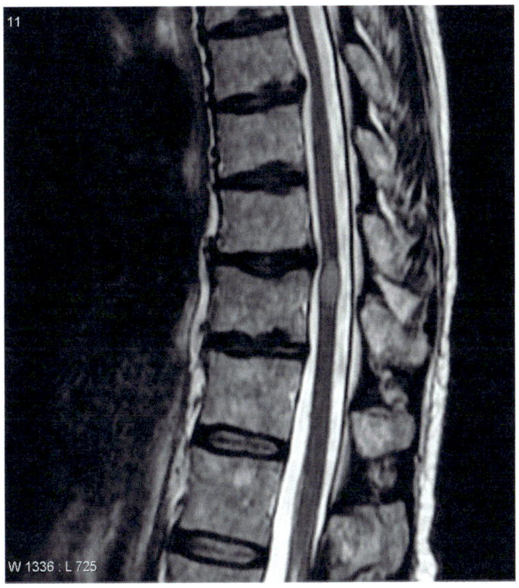

Figure 1.9 Neuromyelitis optica

Source: https://upload.wikimedia.org/wikipedia/commons/d/de/Transverse_myelitis_MRI.jpg,*Creative Commons License.*

These non-HLA genes are involved in the production of cytokines, adaptive immunological responses, and innate immunity. These genes also control the growth of B and T cells. Many single nucleotide polymorphisms (SNPs) in non-HLA genes have also been related to

SSc, according to the genome-wide analysis. Studies on microRNA (miRNA) expression in SSc have also revealed associations between other miRNAs, such as epidermal growth factor.

1.6 Neurological diseases

As the population ages, neurological diseases become more prevalent. Many neurological conditions, including multiple sclerosis, Alzheimer's disease, neuromyelitis optica (Figure 1.9), Parkinson's disease, and myasthenia gravis, have immunogenetic bases (foundations). Parkinson's disease and multiple sclerosis serve as models to illustrate how immunogenetics affects neurological conditions. A prominent cause of non-traumatic neurological impairment in the young population is multiple sclerosis (MS), an inflammatory and possibly incapacitating disease of the central nervous system. The pathophysiology of this disease is significantly influenced by ethnicity and family history. MS is a complex disease that is influenced by both heredity and the environment. MS was among the first diseases to be linked to HLA. The immune system attacks (targets) the myelin sheath that envelops the axons and facilitates communication between the brain and the rest of the body. Mostly involving HLA class II components, MS is likely one of the earliest genetic diseases where HLA connection has been observed. MS is seen as an autoimmune disease in which CD^{+} autoreactive T cells, th1 cell polarization, and CD^{8+} T cells are excited and can damage CNS or central nervous system tissues(Sinha et al., 2014). One hundred genetic loci have been linked to multiple sclerosis. Roughly 10% of genetic alterations are caused by HLA. The most common and progressing neurodegenerative disease is Parkinson's disease (PD). It has been demonstrated to have an immunogenetic foundation, just as other neurological disorders. Inflammation is the primary characteristic of Parkinson's disease. This disease is characterized by increased activation of major histocompatibility class II expression. Parkinson's disease is not a single disease but rather presents a variety of clinical and genetic subgroups (types). Nearly 10% of cases are monogenic, but 90% of cases are multifactorial, with a variety of environmental factors contributing to the disease. It is an extremely complex disease. Two of the 41 loci linked to Parkinson's disease are located inside the HLA locus, which codes for genes like MHC II. The combination of genetic analysis and immunological data suggests that immunogenetics plays a significant role in this disease. Immunogenetics is crucial to the etiology of neurological disorders.

1.7 Infectious diseases

Infectious diseases are the most prevalent health problems. A multitude of genetic factors, in addition to environmental factors, are crucial in the etiology of certain diseases, such as tuberculosis, hepatitis B virus (HBV), HIV, and HCV infections. Prolonged viral infections have a substantial impact on the immune system. Individuals with infections such as HCV/HIV have immune system defects, including weakened CD^{4+} and CD^{8+} T cells, which makes it harder for them to fight off the infection. In terms of TB, it is an infectious disease caused by *Mycobacterium tuberculosis* (MTb)(P. L. Lin & Flynn, 2015).

BCG is the only vaccine that is officially known to provide protection against this disease. Interferons were thought to be innate inflammatory cytokines and potent mediators between innate and adaptive immunity long before it was discovered that they might have some antiviral qualities. In addition to environmental variables, immunogenetics has been identified to have a role in the etiology of this disease. It has been discovered that

TLRs, C-type lectin receptors or CLRs, and NLRs are among the innate immune receptors that may identify MTb. HLA genes and non-HLA genes are examples of genetic factors. HLA-Dr1 and HLA-DQ1 antigens have been linked to TB susceptibility. Immunogenetics plays a significant influence in the development of HIV, another viral disease. It has been discovered that there is phenomenological genetic variability in HIV. The host genetic factors are linked to both the probability of viral infection and the resistance to HIV infection among exposed individuals. They are also one of the elements of the inter-individual variation observed in reactivity to HIV infection. HLA class I genes are among the genetic variations that play a key part in HIV infection. They show the highest correlation (or association), suggesting that CD^{8+} T cells play a vital role in viral resistance. Because HLA proteins give cytotoxic lymphocytes to immunodominant HIV epitopes, they are essential for T cell-mediated adaptive immunity. By interacting with natural killer (NK) cell immunoglobulin-like receptors, HLA contributes to natural killer cell-mediated innate immunity against HIV.

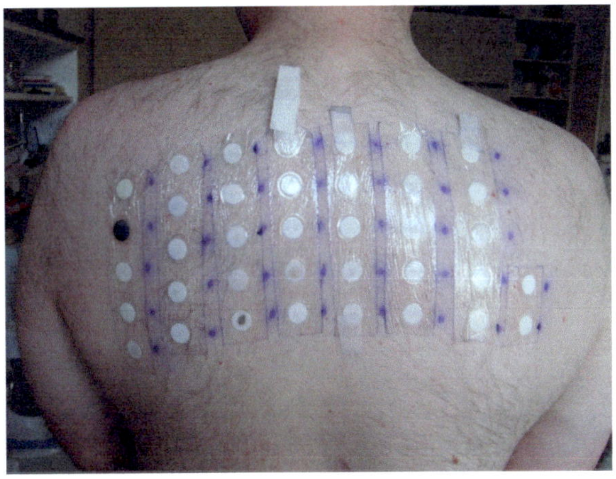

Figure 1.10 Allergic rhinitis

Source: https://upload.wikimedia.org/wikipedia/commons/4/4c/Epikutanni-test.jpg,*Creative Commons License.*

1.8 Immunogenetics of infections

It has also been discovered that HBV and HCV infections have a genetic basis. Immunogenetics contributes to the pathophysiology of these infections. The immune system is compromised as a result of these infections. It has been discovered that both HLA and non-HLA genes have functions. MICA and DEPDC5 are the two genes linked to these infections(Al-Anazi et al., 2014). Allergic rhinitis (Figure 1.10), Asthma, and atopic dermatitis (Figure 1.11) are only a few of the atopic conditions that have recently been linked to immunogenetics.

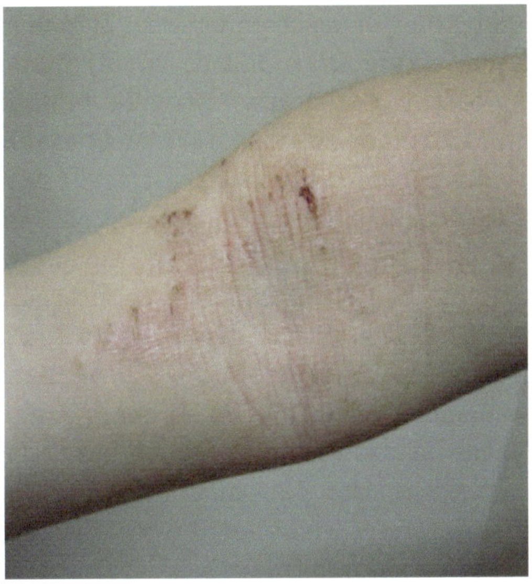

Figure 1.11 Atopic dermatitis

Source: https://upload.wikimedia.org/wikipedia/commons/1/1a/Atopy2010.JPG,*Creative Commons License.*

Th2-mediated processes are the cause of several categories of diseases known as atopic diseases. Th2 cytokines stimulate IgE^{+} memory B cells and plasma cells to produce more IgE. The majority of these atopic diseases have genes on chromosome 6 that also contain MHC genes. These atopic disorders are genetically similar to other autoimmune disorders. T cell-driven inflammation and a strong genetic predisposition are features of atopic dermatitis(Werfel et al., 2016). Multiple immunological mechanisms have been linked with this disease. The emphasis on immunogenetic research was established by Landsteiner's discovery of antigenic variations in human blood and Bernstein's discovery of the genetic regulation of the A-B-O blood types. Irwin coined the term immunogenetics in 1936 to describe his studies on red cell antigens in dove hybrids.

The discovery by Heidelberger and Avery that carbohydrates were necessary for immunological methods to identify different types of pneumococci marked a turning point in our understanding of the chemical basis of biological accuracy or precision. It was widely believed that proteins could only provide biological specificity before this discovery. Most attempts to isolate serum proteins from closely similar species were unsuccessful. Research on human and animal blood types, or red cell antigens, dominated the field of immunogenetics. On the other hand, it was found that some red cell antigens were important in the transplantation experiments in mice. Some researchers proposed the terms histocompatibility genes and antigens to determine the genomes and pathogens necessary for graft function during the grafting of a skin or an organ.

These genes are now viewed as belonging to a gene cluster called the System of Histocompatibility Genes (SHG) or Major Histocompatibility Gene Complex (MHC)(Reith & Mach, 2001). This area of immunogenetics gained prominence and is today a major component of human medicine. Due to the serological methods, antigenic markers are found in soluble plasma components. The study of antigenic variations in plasma proteins was advanced by immunodiffusion and immunoelectrophoretic techniques, and the term allotypes was first used by Oudin to refer to specific genetic variations among organisms.

1.9 HLA gene regulation

Understanding the genetic regulation of immunoglobulin chain formation and association has also been advanced by allotype research. Some researchers established a novel field of immunogenetics by employing simple synthetic polypeptides with minimal structural variation as immunogens. They found that unique immune response (It) genes governed the recognition of particular antigens. Some scientists demonstrated that general immunological resistance was a polygenic characteristic by genetically modifying mice for elevated/low susceptibility to a dynamic multideterminant immunogen. The surfaces of almost every animal cell contain histocompatibility antigens. The use of lymphocytes for serological identification is common. Since histocompatibility antigens were initially discovered in mice, inbred mouse strains were a useful model for researching histocompatibility antigens in other species. Antigens from the H-2 system comprise the major histocompatibility complex (MHC) in mice. The MHC mechanism, which is comparable to the H-2 system, is present in nearly all species. The MHC is a complex genetic system located on chromosome 6 (short arm) that spans approximately 4 Mb. Human leukocyte antigen (HLA) loci are crucial for transplant compatibility because they mostly code for antigens that express on the nucleated cell surface. The immune response is regulated by HLA molecules, which distinguish between self and non-self. They are found in immunoglobulins, CD4, CD8, T cell receptors, and other immunoglobulin supergene family molecules. T cells are presented with the antigen via HLA molecules, which activate an immunological reaction. When agglutinating antibodies were found in the sera of multiparous women and polytransfused individuals in the 1950s, the HLA mechanism was identified(Muzaffer et al., 2022). The receptive structures of such sera showed that they did not respond to autologous responses and only recognized cells from distinct individuals, suggesting that agglutinins were alloreactive and detected antigens at the polymorphic gene level. HLA laboratories must routinely sample and track the serum of potential HLA antibody recipients in accordance with standard protocol for antibody screening.

1.10 Other research findings

Genes that regulate the synthesis of cytokines, heat shock proteins, complement system proteins, and the immune response-related enzyme 21-OH hydroxylase are found in the Class III MHC. The three parts of the HLA molecule are intracellular, intramembranous, and extracellular. The extracellular area is divided into three sections by the peptide-binding domains alpha 1 and 2, which correspond to alleles in the second and third exons of the gene, respectively.

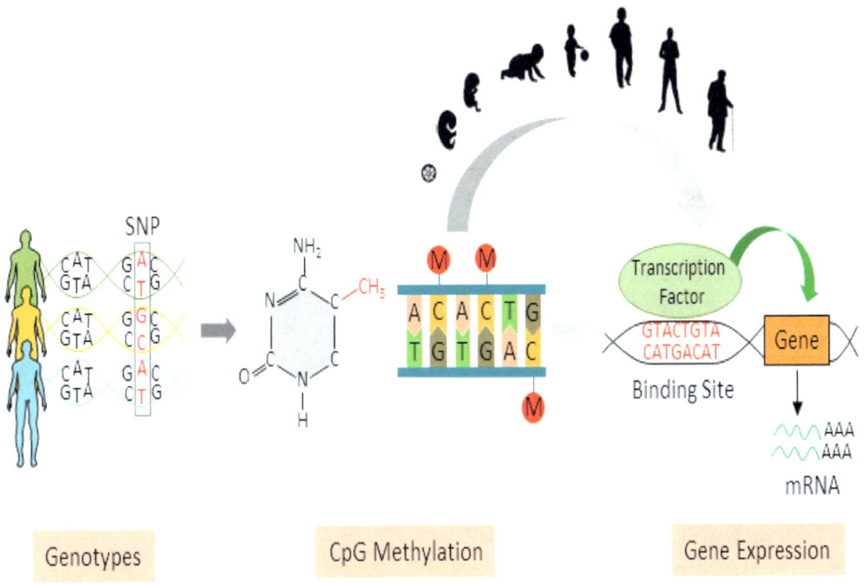

Figure 1.12 Single nucleotide polymorphisms

Source: https://upload.wikimedia.org/wikipedia/commons/1/1e/Associations_between_SNPs%2C_methylation_patterns_and_gene_expression.png,*Creative Commons License.*

These antigenic peptide domains are bound by the HLA Class I antigen, which then interacts with a range of T cell receptors(Bentley & Mariuzza, 1996). HLA Class II was discovered as a result of the activation of lymphocytes from HLA-identical individuals in mixed lymphocyte cultures. HLA Class II antigens are only carried by immune cells such as B lymphocytes, activated T lymphocytes, and macrophages. Three separate types of human Class II molecules i.e., HLA-DQ, HLA-Dr, and HLA-DP are encoded by genes located in various locations and have varying numbers of alpha and beta chain alleles. HLA typing is presently performed on the beta chain because it is even more pleiotropic than the alpha chain. Two extracellular domains, alpha 1 and 2, with oligosaccharide binding sites, are present in the alpha chain (hydrophilic region); similarly, the beta chain (hydrophilic) section or fragment has two extracellular domains, beta 1 and 2(Hohenester & Engel, 2002). The second and third exons are linked to the first (alpha 1 + beta 1) and second (alpha 2 + beta 2) extracellular hydrophilic domains, respectively, according to the amino acid sequences, which show that the initial extracellular domains of both chains are complicated. The distribution of distinct haplotypes and alleles varies among populations and ethnic groups. Most unique alleles are only found in exons that indicate domains of antigen-presenting cells; however, some mutations are found in introns or exons in other domains. In some instances, the amino acid sequence remains unchanged whereas the change only occurs in the nucleotide sequences. The degree of allele description in HLA typing depends on the quantity and type of probes or primers utilized for the analysis. High resolution typing requires a combination of primers or probes and a number of methods to address the common HLA ambiguities. A computer software is required to to evaluate and assign HLA alleles and correlate the results with the dataset of WHO-recognized alleles. For hematopoietic stem cell transplantation to be successful, the donor and patient must be histocompatible. Determination at the antigen level is typically adequate in organ transplantation and can be accomplished by molecular biology or serological methods.

1.11 SNP analyses

Single nucleotide polymorphisms (Figure 1.12) or SNPs include substitutions, deletion insertion polymorphisms or DIPs, and short tandem repeats or STRs. Multibase variability includes inversions, additional repeats, insertion deletions (INDELs), etc. When creating the first genetic and physical map of the human genome, STRs and SNPs were very helpful as genetic markers. The sub-microscopic structural genetic polymorphism is gaining acceptance. It includes translocations larger than 1 kb in size, segmental duplications, inversions, and copy number variations. Many of these variants may have functional significance, such as CNV-507 and CNV-505, which share susceptibility loci for psoriasis and sarcoidosis(Redon et al., 2006). Both the complement area and the HLA-DRB1 region, which are specific to particular allelic combinations or haplotypes, are impacted by segmental duplications. Enzyme-linked immunosorbent assay (ELISA) was the first assay to use antigenic determinants. Some methods rely on soluble or recombinant HLA molecules attached to polystyrene units and are now thought to be the appropriate standard for antibody assessment and recognition. Luminex analysis, on the other hand, uses globules that are distinguished by changes in their primary fluorescent dyes. HLAs are used to treat particular groups of gobbets. These clusters of globules are accumulated in one well to carry out several tests.

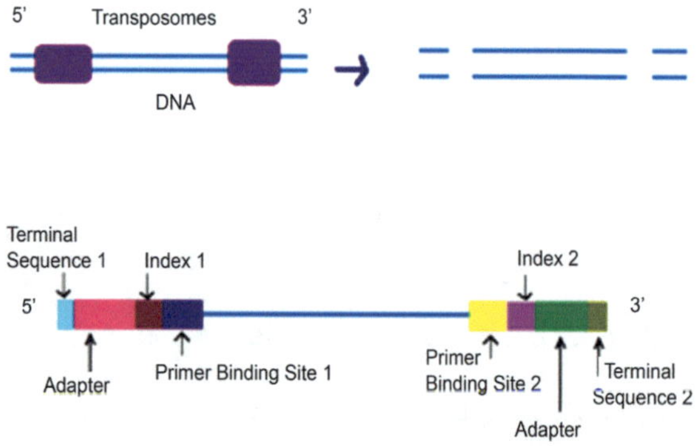

Figure 1.13 PCR-based sequencing

Source: By DMLapato - Own work, CC BY-SA 4.0, https://commons.wikimedia.org/w/index.php?curid=43778910,*Creative Commons License.*

The current technique for determining HLA genes in advance is PCR-sequence-based typing (Figure 1.13), or PCR-SBT. Another technique is

Sanger sequencing, which is utilized in bleach terminator interaction and is also frequently utilized in automated equipment for repetitive HLA typing. Sanger created a DNA sequencing method that uses ddNTP (di-deoxynucleotides) as a substrate(Gaastra & Oudega, 1983). When combined at the 3' termination end of the developing sequence, the chain becomes clogged, especially at the nitrogen bases, because the sequence lacks a 3'-hydroxyl assembly. When activated by a laser, each of the four distinct bleaches that are used to identify the additional feedback of the nitrogen bases A, C, G, and T releases its bright distinct wavelength. Chain elongation ends and diverse deoxyribose nucleic acid fragments of varying sizes are created as a result of the random assimilation of the dNTP. After PCR sequencing, these DNA fragments are separated via capillary duct electrophoresis. The distinct fluorescence emitted allowed for the identification and differentiation of each of the four nitrogen bases at the fragment ends. A catalog that includes all of the configurations of known genes is used to assess the nucleotide sequences produced by sequence analysis tools. Different gene magnitudes with distinctive locations, such as exon 2 for HLA class II and exons 2 and 3 for HLA class I, are suppressed during sequencing for HLA resolutions. Sequence-based typing (SBT), which is regulated by obscurities, is an important method for expressing HLA genes and may also be used to categorize unknown genes. This requires two or more allele arrangements because many HLA alleles may share the same characteristics.

1.12 Gestational immunity

The self/nonself immune recognition hypothesis and the identification of the major histocompatibility complex (MHC) suggested that lymphocytes have receptors for allogeneic cells and nonself antigens, which causes the allograft to be rejected. This model of transplantation immunology was also relevant to gestational immunology. When recipient T cells recognize donor MHC molecules as nonself, acute graft rejection takes place. At first, several ideas suggested that this phenomenon did not occur during pregnancy or that the mother's immune system was continuously suppressed. However, the later discoveries of antigen-specific T cells in the fetus and antibody-facilitated reactions in the mother cannot be explained by this mechanism. The adaptive immunological environment inhibits antigen-specific immunity following implantation. Regulatory T cells (Treg) mediate this tolerance. Treg cells reduce inflammatory responses by acting as potent mediators between natural killer (NK) cells, macrophages, dendritic cells (DCs), and elements of innate and adaptive immunity. The interactions between HLA molecules and ligands that take place at the placenta, the fetomaternal interface, are the main focus of gestational immunity. The placenta's development and function can impact the fetus's growth, development, and survival as well as the mother's immune response. After fertilization, the outer layer of cells, known as trophectoderm, develops the placenta, while the inner layer, known as the blastocyst, forms the embryo. Modifications to the endometrial stroma cell morphology, remodeling of the mother spiral arteries, and immune cell infiltration and activity are all necessary for decidualization. Immune response cells comprise about 45% of the decidual cells. NK cells make up 66% of them, followed by macrophages (25%), T cells (10%), B cells, and DCs, which are much less common(Yang et al., 2011). The EVTs (Extra villous trophoblast) may come into direct contact with the immune cells at the myometrium and decidua. Loss of pregnancy may arise from major repercussions such as immune cell rejection at the site of implantation or signal pathway blockage.

The placenta serves as a barrier during fetal growth, inhibits contact with the fetus's somatic cells, restricts the contact of the mother's immune cells to the trophoblast, fosters an anti-inflammatory environment, permits tolerance, and makes it easier to avoid the mother's immune responses. The placenta does not, however, offer a comprehensive immune barrier. When the mother's blood is present at the intervillous spot (site), the villous trophoblast cells merge to form syncytiotrophoblasts or ST. Anti-HLA alloantibodies may form as a result of syncytial cells entering the bloodstream as soluble fetal antigens. A mechanism known as fetal microchimerism allows trophoblast cells to be injected into the mother's circulation, effectively resulting in a type of genetic sharing. Similarly, maternal microchimerism, which is observed in nearly 40% of healthy pregnancies, can also happen when maternal immune cells and platelets are present in umbilical cord blood. EVT and chorionic HLA class I and II expressions are regulated during pregnancy, and this is important for a healthy pregnancy outcome. T cells are unable to recognize and adhere to the placenta because the villous ST does not express any HLA I or II molecules. The placenta is effectively protected from the immune cells of the mother by this protecting mechanism. The EVT cannot function as an antigen-presenting cell or cause maternal T cells to recognize it because it only expresses HLA class I. Despite having IFN gamma receptors, trophoblasts are unable to express HLA class II antigens, which prevents them from starting the transduction pathway.

The expression of HLA-B antigens and the absence of HLA class II and HLA-A molecules on EVT inhibit the maternal T cell alloimmune response to paternal-derived HLA antigens. The presence of HLA-C, HLA-E, and HLA-G molecules further inhibits the damage to EVT by NK cells and T cells(Crespo et al., 2017). Decidual natural killer or dNK cells, which can identify the expression of Killer cell Ig-like receptors (KIRs), specifically recognize the HLA-C1 on extravillous trophoblast (EVT). The presence of haplotype KIR B protects against pregnancy-related problems, whereas its absence increases the risk. The activating KIR2DS1 receptor on the KIR B haplotype interacts with its ligand on NK cells to release cell-mediated immune molecules that cause placental trophoblast invasion. However, if the fetus has an additional copy of HLA-C2 and is born to homozygous KIR A mothers, such as when the mother is C1/C2 and the baby is C2/C2, or if the second allele is of paternal origin, pregnancy complications rise. When maternal uterine NK cells with KIR2DL1 receptors connect with fetal trophoblast HLA-C2, an inhibitory pathway is triggered, which results in a substantial rejection of the placenta and pregnancy-related problems. In addition to the KIR-HLA C interaction, decidual NK cells also use another inhibitory mechanism. The binding of the NKG2D receptor with ligands UL-16 proteins (ULBPs) and MHC class I chain associated proteins A/B causes the cytotoxicity of NK cells at the fetal-maternal interface. This binding triggers the cytotoxic pathway mediated by perforin, which kills the contaminated cells. By preserving maternal tolerance during pregnancy, HLA-G plays a vital role in the fetus' survival and development. HLA-G antigens are expressed by embryonic trophoblast cells from the start of the first trimester. The interaction of the HLA-G protein with decidual immune cells at the feto-maternal interface results in fetal tolerance by preventing $CD8^+$ T lymphocytes and NK cells from cytotoxically attacking the fetus. This results in B cell activity, Treg cell stimulation, and $CD4^+$ T cell inhibition. HLA-G $\alpha 1$ domain interacts with immune cell inhibitory receptors to mediate its immunosuppressive effect(Tronik-Le Roux et al., 2022). While ILT 2 is expressed by $CD8^+$ T cells, $CD4^+$ T cells, monocytes, macrophages, and DCs and interacts with heterodimers of HLA-G, the ILT 4 receptor, which is expressed by macrophages, DCs, and monocytes, interacts with monomeric HLA-G molecules. Trogocytosis is the process by which HLA-G negative cells, such as NK cells, engage with trophoblast cells that express HLA-G, causing the negative immune cells to acquire HLA-G and become positive HLA-G cells. Trogocytosis (Figure 1.14) is a process by which surface molecules are moved from one cell to another through cell-to-cell contact. Once HLA-G is acquired, these negative immune cells produce an environment that suppresses the immune system. Decidual NK cell trogocytosis of HLA-G aids in NK cell preservation of tolerance and immunological function throughout pregnancy.

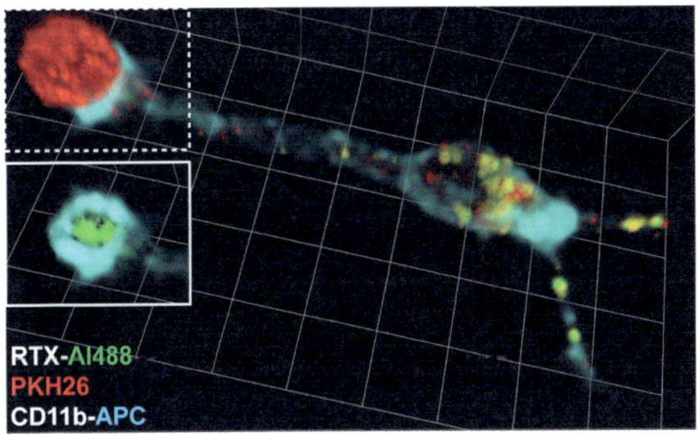

Figure 1.14 Trogocytosis

Source: https://upload.wikimedia.org/wikipedia/commons/a/a8/Ramos_cell_trogocytosis.png,*Creative Commons License.*

The fetal placenta and maternal decidua combine to form the feto-maternal interface. The uterine endometrium is used to create the decidua, which is only generated during pregnancy and sheds at the end of the pregnancy or parturition. Both the fetal and maternal spiral arteries are remodeled during the decidua development process to ensure that the placenta receives a steady supply of maternal blood, allowing for the exchange of waste products, nutrients, and gases. Following implantation, invasive fetal placental trophoblasts implant a fibrinoid layer after the endothelial cells in spiral arteries sheds. Following the blastocyst implantation in the endometrium, the trophoblasts start to infiltrate the uterine spiral artery and endometrial tissue. Maternal lymphocytes, such as $CD4^+$ T cells, $CD8^+$ T cells, and CD^{16} - CD^{56} NK cells, exhibit activation markers on their surface, suggesting that they are able to identify trophoblasts(Saito et al., 2007). A tolerogenic environment is produced at the fetal-maternal interface by trophoblast-derived chemicals and maternal immune response. In this process, maternal leukocytes are essential. Fetal trophoblasts and maternal leukocytes dilate the spiral arteries as a result of these activities, which reduce force and maximize the volume of maternal blood that reaches the placenta. By the third week of pregnancy, villi have formed the placenta. On the outermost surface of the placenta villous tree, a single layer of syncytial syncytiotrophoblasts or SYN lines forms the primary cellular barrier between the fetus and maternal blood. The undifferentiated mononucleated cytotrophoblasts (CTBs) are found beneath the SYN layer. These CTBs are precursor trophoblasts found at the tips of the anchoring villi that can either differentiate into mononucleated EVTs or merge to replenish the SYN layer. The placental primary endocrine component, the SYN layer, produces the hormones progesterone and human chorionic gonadotropin (hCG). Along with the flow of gases and waste products across the maternal-fetal interface, it also promotes the exchange of nutrients.

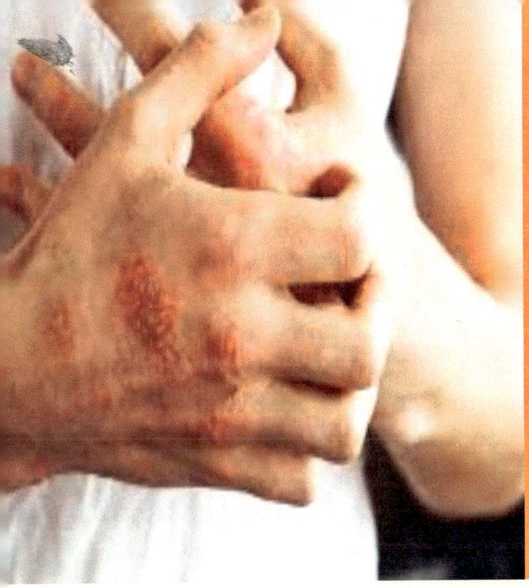

Chapter 2

INTRODUCTION TO AUTOIMMUNE DISEASES

Contents

2.1 Introduction

An autoimmune disease is a condition in which autoimmunity either directly causes the disease or significantly contributes to it. It relies on immunological effector systems that have the capacity to damage host cells. The effector mechanisms, which include soluble antibodies, $CD4^+$ T cells, $CD8^+$ T cells, macrophages, and other phagocytic cells and mast cells, are identical to those linked to previous immune responses to infections(Averbeck et al., 2007). An antibody can cause damage by generating harmful immune complexes, blocking or stimulating a receptor, or directly attaching to a cellular antigen and activating the complement system. The receptors for the Fc portion of the antibody can modify the course of autoimmune and immunological responses in different ways. Since antibodies appear to be unable to reach the intracellular antigen in sufficient numbers, $CD4^+$ and $CD8^+$ T lymphocytes (Figure 2.1) are frequently associated with diseases. However, it is often challenging to distinguish between the contributions of cell-mediated damage and antibody-mediated damage in human autoimmune diseases.

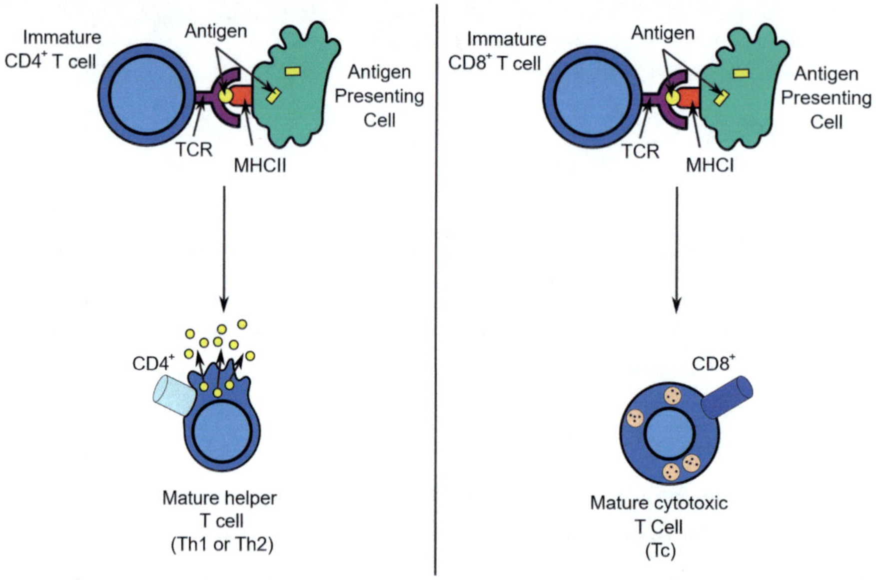

Figure 2.1 $CD4^+$ and $CD8^+$ T lymphocytes

Source: https://upload.wikimedia.org/wikipedia/commons/4/4d/Antigen_presentation.svg,Creative Commons License.

It is important to keep in mind that B cells contribute to the harmful autoimmune process by producing antibodies as well as acting as highly efficient antigen-capturing cells and APCs, especially for activated/memory T cells. Autoimmune disease is linked to a combination of environmental exposure, genetic predisposition, and a substantial amount of chance. Random receptor mutations, somatic mutations, and environmental impacts are some of the mechanisms that could lead to chance events. Research studies have acknowledged the significance of heredity in autoimmune disease, with comparisons of genetically identical and non-identical twins revealing higher rates in the former and familial aggregations of autoimmune diseases. Animals can be inbred to develop autoimmune diseases on their own, and an increasing number of susceptibility genes are being found and their roles explained (linked). According to some studies, susceptibility alleles at the MHC class II locus are the main causes of autoimmune disorders.

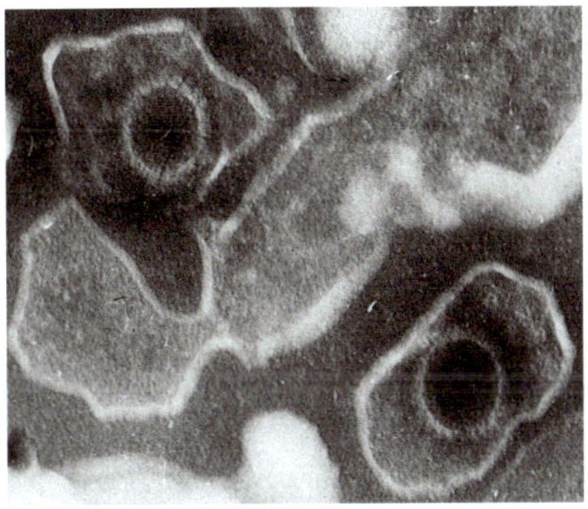

Figure 2.2 Epstein-Barr herpes type virus

Source: https://upload.wikimedia.org/wikipedia/commons/0/07/Epstein_Barr_Virus_virions_EM_10.1371_journal.pbio.0030430.g001-L.JPG,Creative Commons License.

2.2 Genes in autoimmune diseases

The AIRE genes and apoptotic genes like Fas and FasL, have been linked to influencing the risk of developing autoimmune disease. Alleles at the CD152 locus or allelic forms of genes or their promoters producing cytokines associated with immune responses are examples of genes that frequently control the immune response(Stojanova et al., 2016). Non-immune genes should also not be ignored. Even while genetic predisposition has been shown to have a part in almost all autoimmune disorders, its overall impact initially appears to be quite minimal because heredity accounts for less than one-third of the chance of producing an autoimmune disease in humans. However, as our understanding of the genome grows, this could alter. The Epstein-Barr herpes type virus (EBV) (Figure 2.2) is of interest because it is also lymphomagenic. Medications (drugs) that mimic the symptoms of traditional autoimmune diseases are among the instances of environmental chemical causation. Two drugs, procainamide, and hydralazine, can cause a lupus-like reaction with all of the serologic concomitants. Their causal role can be demonstrated by the fact that stopping the drug causes complete remission and that the autoimmune state returns more quickly. Due to the stochastic processes that are essential to producing the diversity of the immune response, identical twins do not have the same immune systems. There are compelling indications that preclinical autoimmunity may remain dormant for long periods and that autoimmune diseases develop gradually. The development of symptoms may be determined by additional environmental triggers and/or random variations. Immune system activation in the absence of an external risk to the organism is a characteristic of a variety of disorders. In these conditions, tissue damage and inflammation happen without infection, exposure to toxins, or tumor formation. These diseases, which include familial Mediterranean fever, atherosclerosis, and Behçet disease, are defined as those that exhibit innate immune system activation and an excess of inflammatory mediators without any indication of an immune response specific to an antigen. In certain diseases, the adaptive immune response is triggered, resulting in T and B cells reacting to self-antigens without any discernible tumor invasion or microbial attack. The adaptive immune system cells interact in a coordinated manner, with dendritic cells (DCs), T cells, and B cells interacting to produce the immune system effector response. DCs stimulate B cells and T cells and T cells stimulate B cells and DCs. T cells are activated by B cells. This cascade results in an immune response that uses a variety of effector mechanisms and can identify a wide range of microbial pathogen epitopes.

2.3 APC dynamics

Antigen-presenting cells (APCs), or DCs, are essential for triggering an immune response(von Bubnoff et al., 2001). They exhibit surface expression of class I major histocompatibility complex (MHC) molecules, which allow T cells to be presented with intracellular antigens, like other cells. DCs contain class II MHC molecules, which allow extracellular antigens to be presented and are found on a small group of cells. Each person (subject) has a distinct collection of MHC molecules since class I and II molecules have many alleles. DCs express a variety of pattern-recognition receptors that bind microbial antigens and nonpolymorphic receptors known as Toll-like receptors (TLRs) (Figure 2.3).

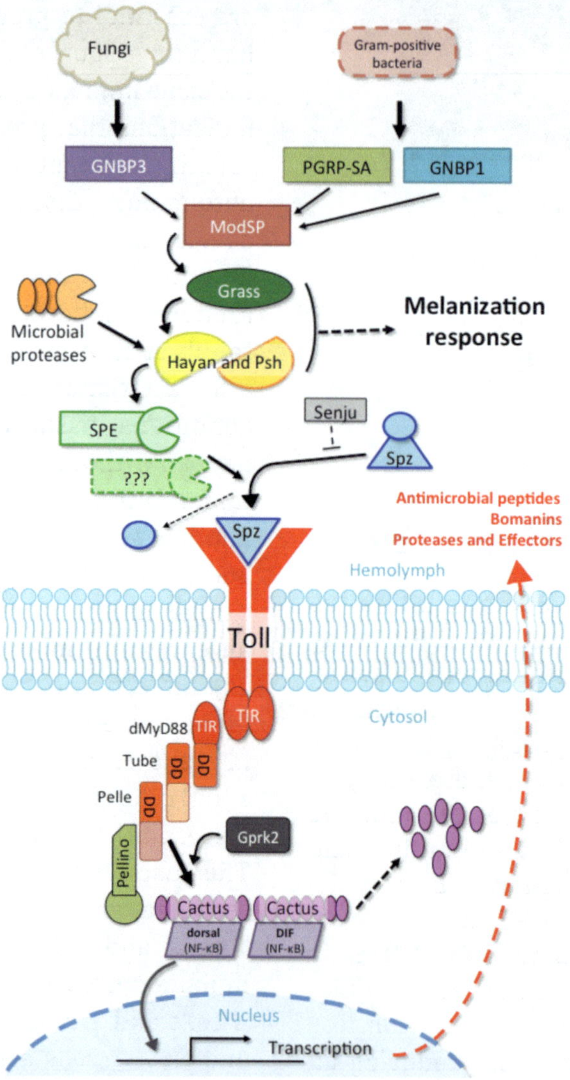

Figure 2.3 Toll-like receptors

Source: https://upload.wikimedia.org/wikipedia/commons/a/a9/Toll_Pathway_of_Drosophila_melanogaster.jpg,Creative Commons License.

The DCs increase the production of costimulatory molecules and provide a necessary signal for activation when these receptors are engaged.

2.4 T and B cells

A wide range of microbial antigens can be recognized and responded to by each DC, which is significant. Every T cell and every B cell expresses a single antigen receptor. There is no inheritance of the T- or B-cell repertoire because these antigen receptors are obtained by gene rearrangements that take place in somatic cells. The thymus is where T lymphocytes develop. A class I or class II MHC molecule linked to a short peptide generated from an intracellular or extracellular protein antigen, respectively, makes up the molecular complex on the surface of an APC that is recognized by a distinct receptor (TCR) expressed by each T cell. Mature T cell activation requires signaling via the TCR and costimulatory molecules. A single antigen receptor is also expressed by B cells; however, the B-cell receptor (BCR) detects native antigens instead of processed antigens. Signaling via the BCR and costimulatory molecules is also necessary for B-cell activation. In addition to secreting antibodies, activated B cells can act as APCs to activate more T cells in the immunological response.

Both T and B cells can multiply in response to antigenic stimulation, which results in the development of cells with a memory phenotype and clonal expansions of cells with distinct antigenic specificity. After being exposed to the antigen again, memory cells respond more quickly and effectively. B cells can experience class switching of the immunoglobulin heavy chain gene and random somatic mutation of the BCR. During an immune response, low-affinity IgM antibodies get converted into high-affinity IgG antibodies. Each person (individual) has their own repertoire of high-affinity IgG-producing B cells, which are reactivated by the memory response. For the immune system to be successful, there must be few cells that react to self-antigens and a sufficient number of T and B cells in both the naïve and memory repertoires that can react to a variety of microbial antigens. T-cell or antibody reactivity to self is the cause of tissue damage in autoimmune disease. Although an infection may trigger immunological activation, it must continue even in the absence of any microbial antigen that can be detected. It is crucial to note that while when anti-self reactivity is present in many conditions classified as autoimmune disorders, there may not be enough proof to conclude that tissue damage is actually caused by self-reactivity. Transferring autoantibodies to a rodent host can occasionally express if they are harmful; however, T-cell reactivity cannot be transferred from humans to rodents since T-cell activation and T-cell effector function only take place in the presence of self-MHC molecules. Therefore, not all autoimmune disorders have been shown to exhibit the toxicity of the autoimmune response. In certain cases, the presence of B and T lymphocytes in the afflicted tissue alone leads to the assumption that the disease has an autoimmune etiology(Nikolajczyk, 2010).

2.5 Autoimmunity

Our knowledge of the pathophysiology of autoimmune diseases has benefited from the use of animal models. Vaccination with a self-antigen can cause certain autoimmune disorders in animals. Although all of the animal models have greatly advanced our knowledge of autoimmunity, it is crucial to acknowledge that their ability to accurately represent human disease is unknown. The effector mechanisms of tissue damage in several of these models might resemble human disease more than the processes of autoreactivity induction. The human disease and animal models of autoantibody-mediated tissue injury are likely similar. It is also important to understand that human diseases can vary and that the animal models we use for intensive research may only represent a portion of people who have a certain disease. Finding animal models that closely resemble human disease and that can explain to us the most about the pathophysiology of disease, genetic susceptibility to disease, and successful treatment is a challenge. The prevalence of all autoimmune diseases is almost 5%, which is remarkable considering that only a small percentage of people are affected by each. Understanding the high prevalence of autoimmune diseases requires knowledge of two crucial things. First, every healthy immune system has autoreactivity. Actually, autoreactivity is used to choose the repertoire of immunocompetent cells that offer protective immunity. The immune system is shaped by the regulation of autoreactivity, which necessitates attention to prevent the development of pathogenic autoreactivity linked to tissue damage.

Target-organ vulnerability is necessary for autoimmune disease in addition to autoreactivity. Recent research on the genetic foundations (basis) of autoimmunity has revealed that the genetic variables influencing autoreactivity and specific organ vulnerability are different. People with various autoimmune diseases may share pathways that promote autoreactivity. Epidemiologic research and investigations of autoimmune disease in animals have demonstrated that almost all autoimmune diseases have a hereditary component. A small number of autoimmune conditions seem to be monogenic. The AIRE gene, which codes for a protein that triggers the expression of tissue-specific genes in medullary epithelial cells in the thymus, is deleted in autoimmune-polyendocrinopathy-candidiasis-ectodermal-dystrophy (APECED), a human autoimmune disease affecting multiple endocrine organs. T cells that react to peptides derived from tissue-specific proteins are subject to negative selection by these cells. A range of autoreactive T cells that develop into immunocompetent cells that orchestrate an immunological attack on different organs are not eliminated when AIRE expression is absent.

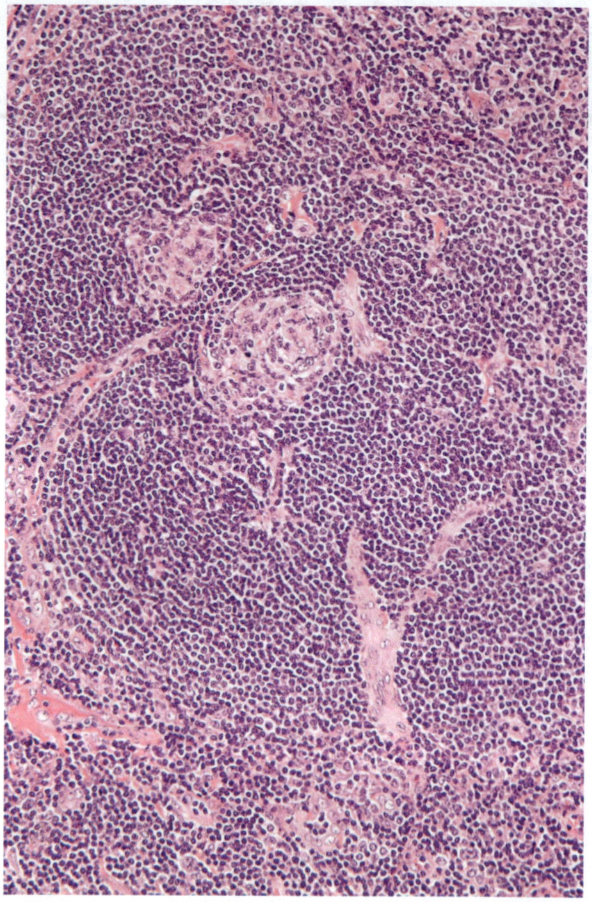

Figure 2.4 Autoimmune lymphoproliferative syndrome

Source: https://upload.wikimedia.org/wikipedia/commons/6/66/Castleman_disease_-_high_mag.jpg,Creative Commons License.

The phenotype of the disease that develops can vary, but it seems that the loss of the AIRE gene is required for autoimmunity. Autoimmunity may result from a mutation in the Fas gene. Activated lymphocytes express the Fas protein(Suda & Nagata, 1997). When the Fas ligand engages Fas, the Fas-expressing cell dies, which is a crucial step in suppressing the immunological response. Autoimmune lymphoproliferative syndrome (ALPS), (Figure 2.4) a condition marked by an excess of T and B cells and the production of autoantibodies, affects people who lack Fas expression. Not every person with impaired Fas expression exhibits ALPS; hence, other genes must also influence the disease phenotype in this condition.

2.6 Susceptibility loci

Multiple susceptibility loci must coexist for a disease phenotype to manifest in the majority of autoimmune disorders. Every locus is an area that has been linked to the disease phenotype by linkage analysis. In mouse models, regions that decrease the autoimmune phenotype have been found in 27 autoimmune diseases. A combination of susceptibility and resistance loci determines an individual's (patient) chance of getting an autoimmune disease. Although genes involved in the cellular processes may exist within the various loci, it is feasible that vulnerability to a certain autoimmune disease may be mediated by completely different sets of genetic loci. The genetic analysis of autoimmune diseases is more difficult. The expression of a specific HLA haplotype is a part of the genetic basis of an autoimmune disease. For instance, in the white population, rheumatoid arthritis is strongly linked to the expression of a group of DR4 alleles with a specific structural motif known as the shared epitope. The same correlation between DR4 alleles and rheumatoid arthritis is not shown in other ethnic groups. As a result, multiple etiopathogenic mechanisms may produce a similar symptom complex. People with reactive arthritis express B27 or, B7 class I MHC molecules(Hermann et al., 1993). Like many other autoimmune disorders, multiple sclerosis, systemic lupus, and diabetes exhibit specific HLA correlations (associations). Although there is the hypothesis that the antigens and antigenic peptides targeted by the autoimmune response are determined by these HLA associations with autoimmune disease, it is also evident that several non-MHC genes within or in linkage disequilibrium with the MHC locus aid in immune response regulation. A genetic predisposition to autoimmunity is influenced by these non-MHC genes.

Many genes within each susceptibility loci contribute to the tendency for autoimmunity, and the majority of susceptibility loci seem to represent extensive disease-related haplotypes. Many genes and loci related to autoimmunity have now been identified. There is increasing evidence that genetic vulnerability may result via gene combinations within each gene locus rather than from a single gene in each locus. Analyzing susceptibility loci in murine models reveals that many genes within each locus influence pathways that support autoimmunity. For instance, systemic lupus erythematosus is linked to autoimmunity through a locus on chromosome 1(Long et al., 2016). Certain Fc receptor gene alleles and non-Fc receptor genes at this locus may be risk factors for the disease. Certain epidemiologic studies have revealed that specific alleles of at least three genes contribute to the autoimmune diathesis in each individual. Autoimmunity risk factors include genes related to lymphocyte survival, activation, and downregulation. Therefore, a malfunction in nearly any process of lymphocyte homeostasis can lead to autoimmunity, and have an impact on thresholds for autoreactive lymphocyte negative selection. It was documented in clinical practice that autoimmune diseases tend to run in families. This scientific basis is now well established; many autoimmune diseases can be influenced by the same susceptibility genes. For instance, the CARD15 (NOD-2) gene is linked to both psoriasis and inflammatory bowel disease, while a polymorphism of CTLA-4, an inhibitory costimulatory molecule found on activated T cells, carries risk for autoimmune hemolytic anemia, insulin-dependent diabetes, and Graves' disease (Figure 2.5). The variations in disease phenotype could be due to related genes, those controlling target organ vulnerability, or those influencing disease severity.

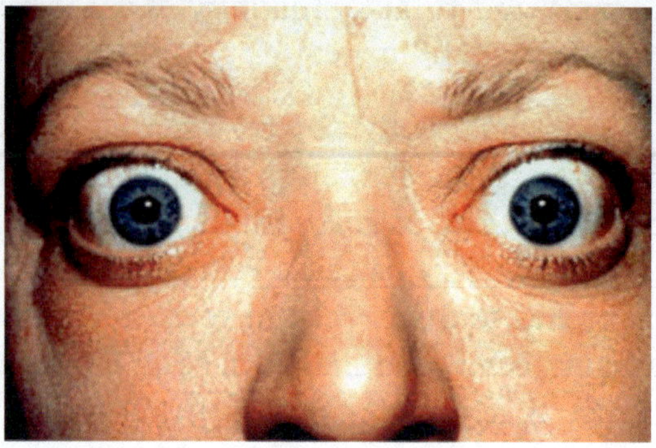

Figure 2.5 Graves' disease

Source: https://upload.wikimedia.org/wikipedia/commons/8/8f/Proptosis_and_lid_retraction_from_Graves%27_Disease.jpg,Creative Commons License.

2.7 Hormones and diseases

Many studies have examined the connection between sex hormones and autoimmune disease because women are more likely than men to develop various autoimmune diseases and to have autoimmunity overall, which is nearly three times more common in women than in men. Making inferences from these investigations has been challenging. Not every autoimmune disease affects women more frequently than men. Certain conditions, including ankylosing spondylitis, are far more common in men. The increased prevalence of disease in women may not always be a result of the impact of female hormones on the immune system because the tendency for autoimmunity can be sex determined or hormonally controlled. The evidence indicates that the effects of sex hormones vary depending on the condition. Estrogen appears to protect against rheumatoid arthritis, despite strong evidence that it can worsen systemic lupus. Target-organ sensitivity to immune-mediated damage or target-organ antigen presentation may be impacted by estrogen or other sex hormones. The association between sex and autoimmunity cannot be explained by a simple pattern. Self-reactive T and B cell activation is a defining feature of autoimmune diseases. The removal of self-reactive immature cells through antigen ligation of the TCR or BCR at crucial developmental stages is a key mechanism of self-tolerance. There must be tolerance in the removal of autoreactive cells for autoimmunity to arise. Autoreactive T and B cells frequently develop because TCRs and BCRs are produced by random gene rearrangements that take place inside the cell nucleus and are not influenced by the self or foreign antigen. T and B cells regularly go through a selection process as they mature in the thymus and bone marrow, the primary lymphoid organs, respectively, to get rid of autoreactive cells and preserve self-tolerance. Since somatic mutation frequently results in autoreactivity, B cells go through a second selection step following somatic mutation of immunoglobulin genes.

2.8 Signal triggers

To obtain the signals required for survival, T cells that grow in the thymus and move into peripheral lymphoid organs must exhibit TCRs with a certain affinity for self-peptide-self-MHC complexes(Ebert et al., 2010). This process is known as positive selection. When thymus-derived T lymphocytes express TCRs with minimal affinity for the self-peptide-self-MHC complexes, they are unable to withstand positive selection and eventually die. The mechanism known as negative selection eliminates T cells that exhibit a high level of reactivity to self-peptide-self-MHC complexes. Each person releases a distinct repertoire of antimicrobial and anti-self-reactive T cells to the periphery, each reflecting a different spectrum of foreign and self-peptide specificities, due to variations in the peptide-MHC complexes found in the thymus and the threshold for negative selection. It is likely that some triggers help save T cells. Similarly, B cells go through negative selection before becoming immunocompetent. Post leaving the bone marrow, B cells migrate as transitional cells in the spleen, where this process continues from the bone marrow. Research is still continuing to determine if B cells must exhibit some level of autoreactivity and undergo positive selection on self-antigen to survive. However, it is evident that self-antigens encountered during early maturation adversely select highly autoreactive B cells, and the threshold for deletion varies from person to person. When BCR cross-linking is strong, the deletion takes place; when it is at its lowest, anergy occurs. As a result, the B-cell repertoire level of autoreactivity varies. In a proinflammatory environment, autoreactive B cells that have been designated to be deleted can be saved by signaling via TLRs or by engaging costimulatory molecules on the B cell membrane. As a result, an individual's repertoire of naïve B cells will change over time, with fewer, lower-affinity autoreactive cells appearing during immunologic quiescence and higher-affinity autoreactive B cells present during infection or inflammation.

2.9 Lymphoid organs

Both the peripheral and primary lymphoid organs experience a negative selection of T and B cells, which enables the thymus and bone marrow to eliminate autoreactive cells that do not come into contact with autoantigen. Peripheral tolerance is the negative selection process. Similar to central tolerance, it is mediated in a non-inflammatory environment by TCR or BCR engagement. While it has long been uncertain whether a deficit in peripheral tolerance in secondary lymphoid organs or in central tolerance in the thymus or bone marrow causes autoimmunity, the current understanding of tolerance induction indicates that this may be a biased distinction. The antigen receptor involvement is essential for both central and peripheral tolerance. People with strong negative selection probably have strong negative selection in both their central and peripheral lymphoid organs, even if several characteristics seem to distinguish central and peripheral tolerance. Similarly, neither central nor peripheral lymphoid organ autoreactive cells can be efficiently deleted by people with tolerance selection. It is evident from animal models that autoimmune disease is caused by poor negative selection in the naïve B- or T-cell repertoire, and that tolerance in negative selection can lead to multiple organ-specific autoimmunity(Romagnani, 2006). The survival and deletion thresholds must be set within reasonable limits. Autoreactivity results from insufficient deletion, while the protective repertoire may be jeopardized by excessive deletion. Any genetic alteration that lessens deletion could increase the likelihood of developing autoimmunity.

2.10 Environmental factors and autoimmunity

Environmental variables can play a vital role in triggering autoimmunity. Smoking, drug use, diet, exposure to chemicals, and solar radiation have all been linked to an increased risk of certain diseases. It is obvious that exposure to antigens or infections can trigger autoimmune disease. The majority of autoimmune disorders may even be the late consequences of an infectious process, according to some theories. The relationship between microbial infection, the antimicrobial response, and autoimmune disease is well-established for certain diseases, such as rheumatic fever. T-cell or antibody cross-reactivity with both microbial and self-antigen has been found for other diseases, and there is suggestive epidemiologic evidence in human or animal models that autoimmunity can occur after microbial infection. Researchers have often tried to link specific infections to the pathophysiology of specific autoimmune diseases, although it is reasonable that many microbial triggers exist for some autoimmune diseases. Both T and B cells must receive two signals to be activated in the periphery: one from the engagement of a costimulatory receptor and the other from the ligation of the antigen receptor. DCs, the crucial APC in a basic immune response, are typically activated when an antigen enters the body. This happens as a result of microorganisms expressing chemicals that attach to the DC pattern-recognition receptors, or TLRs. The costimulatory molecules $CD8^0$ and $CD8^6$ are upregulated on DCs as a result of this interaction, and the DC changes from resting or tolerogenic to active or immunogenic. T cells will be activated if they identify the microbial peptide in either class I or class II MHC molecules on the immunogenic DC(Robinson & Delvig, 2002).

2.11 Autoreactivity

Since all T cells have some degree of autoreactivity when a foreign peptide-self-MHC complex activates a T cell, the activated T cell may also identify a self-peptide-self-MHC complex. The memory T cells can be activated by a lower affinity interaction with the TCR than is necessary to activate initial T cells. Therefore, once a T-lymphocyte develops into a memory T-cell, it may be activated by a self-peptide-self-MHC complex that did not activate it when it was still a naïve cell. Thus, memory T cells may be autoreactive in a proinflammatory environment. Many examples of T-cells generated from autoimmune disease patients that can identify both a self-peptide and a microbial peptide can be found in many research works. This cross-reactivity, which is known as molecular mimicry, is one way that infection might cause autoimmunity. Tolerance in the selection of the naïve T-cell repertoire can be a significant contributor to autoimmunity, as suggested by the concept that molecular mimicry influences autoimmunity, which is evidently valid in rat models of autoimmune disease. Multiple T cells that can be activated by a foreign antigen and exhibit pathogenic autoreactivity are found in those with limited negative selection. When B cells come into contact with microbial antigens, the activated T cell gives them T-cell help or costimulatory signals(Lemoine et al., 2011). B cells that bind both microbial antigen and self-antigen will phagocytose, process, and deliver self-antigen epitopes, which T cells can subsequently detect. B cells can present new self-antigen epitopes and activate T cells with new auto-specificities because they frequently process antigens to distinct peptides than do DCs. Because they stimulate a wider range of T cells, these cross-reactive B cells will hence contribute to a cascade of autoreactivity. Thus, the T-cell repertoire is significantly influenced by the B-cell repertoire. T cells are presented with limited self-antigen when there are fewer autoreactive B cells.

2.12 Clonal growth

Many of the cells that have undergone clonal growth or expansion must be downregulated or eliminated after an immune response is triggered. One important finding on autoimmune diseases is that a malfunction in immunological homeostasis restoration or immune response downregulation may be a risk factor for autoimmunity. The process of developing an immune response to a foreign antigen frequently results in the generation of anti-self responses since all reactivity with foreign antigens also involves reactivity to self-antigen. Each person will have a different level of potential pathogenicity from their autoimmune response.

The same mechanisms that suppress the immune response also suppress autoreactivity, and even potentially harmful autoreactivity is suppressed. As soon as B and T cells are activated, they frequently exhibit downregulation. The BCR and FcRIIB are cross-linked by antigen-antibody complexes, which plays a role in this process for the B cell (Wetzler & Guttormsen, 2004). Autoantibody synthesis is poorly regulated when FcRIIB is missing or insufficient. Activated T cells express several coinhibitory substances. An inhibitory signal is transduced to the T cells upon interaction with their receptors, regulating them to downmodulate their response.

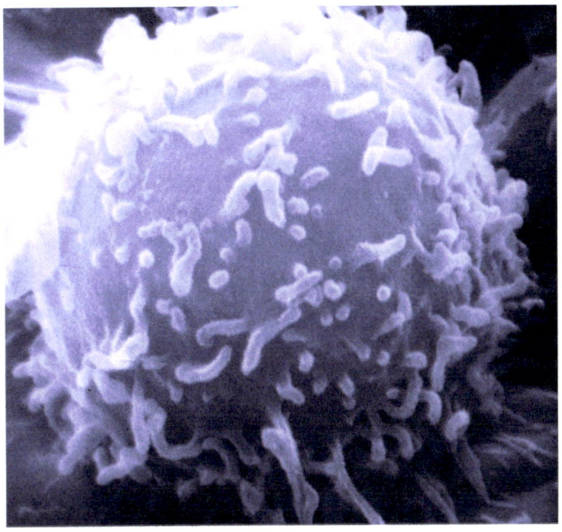

Figure 2.6 Natural killer (NK) T lymphocytes

Source: https://upload.wikimedia.org/wikipedia/commons/8/89/SEM_Lymphocyte.jpg,Creative Commons License.

There is evidence that the T-cell coinhibitory molecule CTLA-4 transduces an inhibitory signal to the APCs when it engages CD80 (B7) on the APC. Many autoimmune disorders are linked to mutations in the coinhibitory molecules PD1 and CTLA-4. Fas-Fas ligand interactions can cause activation-induced cell death in both B and T cells. When this procedure is defective, autoimmunity may result. Controlling the immune response, which is regulated by several inhibitory pathways, is therefore essential to maintaining the immune system's normal homeostasis. A malfunction in the regulation of immunological activation may be a factor in autoimmune disease in certain people. Characterizing and understanding the mechanisms of action of populations of regulatory cells is important.

2.13 Regulatory cells

Lipid antigens in CD1 molecules are recognized by natural killer (NK) T lymphocytes (Figure 2.6). In certain diseases, there is evidence that a decline in this population occurs before autoimmunity manifests. There is evidence linking the development of disease to a shift in this cytokine profile, namely a decrease in the generation of interleukin (IL)-4. It has been demonstrated that using a synthetic ligand to activate NK T cells can stop diabetes in the non-obese diabetic (NOD) animal model(Lin et al., 2009). The thymus contains a population of $CD4^{+}/CD25^{+}$ T cells, which seem to play a key role in the suppression of autoimmunity. These cells can be demarcated from activated T cells that also express CD25 by their expression of the transcription factor Foxp3 and the cell surface receptor GITR. They may also inhibit APCs; they reduce effector T cells in a cell contact-dependent but non-antigen-specific method. In NOD mice, it has been shown that their numbers decrease before they exhibit diabetes and that infusing these cells can postpone diabetes. A population of CD8 suppressor cells has been found in other research studies; these cells may emit immunosuppressive cytokines or directly lyse autoreactive cells. Under specific circumstances of antigen exposure, cells expressing the immunosuppressive cytokines transforming growth factor or IL-10 emerge and, once activated, cause nonantigen-specific suppression. Activating Th2 cells can reduce autoimmunity in murine models, regardless of whether T cells or antibodies are responsible for the tissue damage. This is because Th2 cells regulate the activation of Th1 cells. There is some proof that Th2 cells are preferentially activated by limited antigen levels. The self-antigen is frequently exposed in small quantities and preferentially activates self-reactive nonpathogenic Th2 cells(Lee et al., 2011).

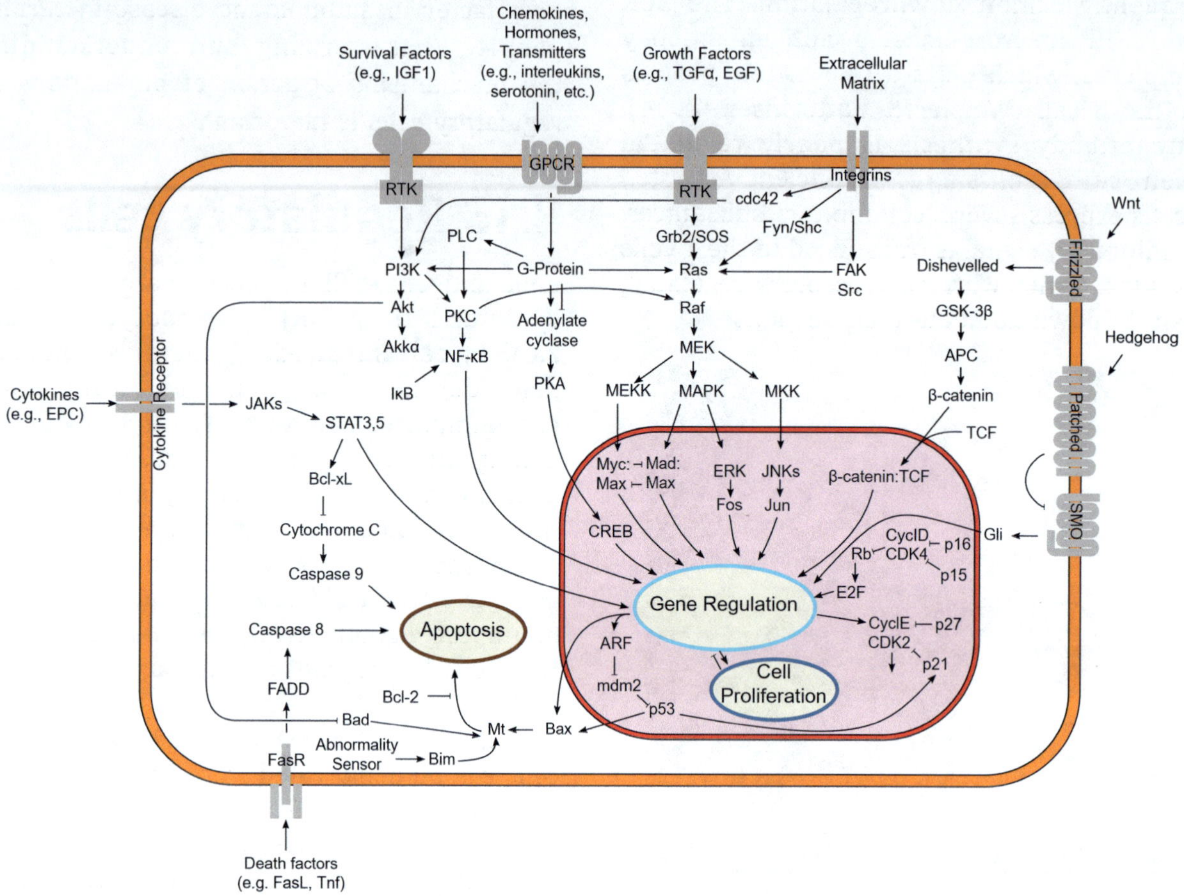

Figure 2.7 Cytokines and their roles

Source: https://upload.wikimedia.org/wikipedia/commons/b/b0/Signal_transduction_pathways.svg,Creative Commons License.

Any one of the several groups of regulatory cells may be lacking in autoimmune diseases. Whether an autoreactive response that develops during microbial exposure is stopped or continues may depend on the ratio of effector cells / regulatory cells. Since both effector and regulatory T cells may become inactive due to severe immunosuppression, novel strategies for treating autoimmunity may focus on figuring out how to restrict effector cells while enabling regulatory cells to proliferate. One of the main questions in autoimmune disease is whether the process is self-driven or antigen-driven, and if the latter, is the antigen foreign or self-antigen. Animal models demonstrate that autoreactivity can be triggered by molecular mimicry after microbial antigen activation. There is evidence that the autoimmune response is triggered by self-antigens. A lupus-like serology with antichromatin reactivity seems to be caused by an overabundance of apoptotic cells. Apoptotic debris can activate B cells, convert tolerogenic DCs into immunogenic APCs, and activate TLRs. A sequestered self-antigen may manifest due to substantial tissue damage. Cell apoptosis after tissue damage may exacerbate the proinflammatory environment. It is obvious that this could trigger an autoimmune reaction. It is crucial to consider whether this reaction is maintained in certain people due to an inadequate return to homeostasis. The autoimmune disease risk factors may also include variations in autoantigens. The extent to which exposure to previously sequestered antigens in an immunogenic environment, abnormal production of autoantigens, or molecular mimicry contribute to disease will become obvious as the genetic vulnerability to autoimmune disease is better investigated.

2.14 Mechanisms

The mechanisms that trigger autoimmune disease may differ significantly from those that spread tissue damage, as studies conducted in the previous years have shown. The cytokine profile of effector cells (Figure 2.7) that migrate into target organs and induce tissue fibrosis may differ from that of autoreactive T and B cells that are activated in 2° lymphoid organs and initiate the disease. It is becoming increasingly evident that the induction of autoreactivity and tissue destruction must be investigated independently at each stage of autoimmune disease, and that the earlier classification of some cytokines as proinflammatory and others as anti-inflammatory may have been inaccurate. Transforming growth factor- β (TGF-β) may speed up tissue fibrosis but slow down the induction of autoreactivity(Li et al., 2006). Similarly, IL-10 inhibits APCs to reduce inflammation at the beginning of the disease, but it can also promote T-cell proliferation, immunoglobulin class switching, and antibody production as the disease progresses. In the early phases of certain autoimmune disorders, even the proinflammatory cytokine interferon-γ can have anti-inflammatory effects. As research on autoimmune diseases advances, it may be crucial to take into account the mechanisms underlying both immune activation and tissue death. It is also crucial to investigate the possibility that cytokines, hormones, or other mediators may have varying impacts on each phase. It is now evident from studies of animal models that disease progression can be manipulated to safeguard (protect) organs from immune-mediated death. Chronic progressive disease activity is represented by the majority of autoimmune disease animal models. When the autoimmune disease starts to show symptoms, it can cause organ failure. On the other hand, a lot of autoimmune diseases in humans are marked by remissions. The cellular processes that result in disease remission are not well understood in human disease. It is also true that not much is understood about what triggers disease flares. Whether flares are a reactivation of dormant memory cells or a de novo activation of naïve autoreactive cells is unknown. Peripheral blood frequently contains insufficient amounts of these cells. They may be so rare that their analysis poses a difficulty, even when they are present in blood and so available for research.

2.15 Dendritic cells

It was discovered that mice spleens included dendritic cells (DCs), which were termed for their branch-like projections. When epidermal Langerhans cells were proven to develop into strong immunostimulatory DCs in vitro, the connection between them and DCs was established. Langerhans cells resemble spleen DCs and gradually increase in stimulatory capability, becoming three to ten times more stimulatory than spleen DCs. Many members of the DC family are found in the majority of bodily tissues and exhibit special qualities not found in other antigen-presenting cells (APCs)(Kashem et al., 2017). T cells specific to harmful antigens previously encountered in the periphery can be sensitized by immature DCs. They serve as a shield for infections in peripheral tissues before migrating to the lymphoid organs, where they activate lymphocytes that are specific to certain microbial antigens and communicate information about the pathogen characteristics and the lymphoid tissues. DCs have strong endocytic activity when they are immature; they have a variety of receptors that are unique to non-self antigens and constitutively macropinocytose extracellular fluids. DCs express the immunogenic class II MHC-peptide complexes only after maturation, rather than presenting antigen right away following absorption. DCs can exhibit antigens encountered earlier in peripheral tissues in the lymphoid organs due to this delay in antigen presentation. As naïve T cells mature, their capacity to process antigens and sensitize them develops sequentially. The synthesis of stimulatory cytokines and the overexpression of costimulatory molecules and MHC restriction elements are linked to this process. DC maturation typically occurs in tandem with their migration to the lymphoid organ T cell-containing zone. The engagement of membrane-bound ligand-receptor pairs necessary for efficient T-cell priming requires the colocalization of fully competent DCs with lymphocytes, which is probably the initial stage of the immune response.

The inflammatory cytokines and microbial components frequently cause DC maturation, which promotes the activation of T cells that are specific for non-self infectious antigens. The Toll-like receptors (TLRs), which identify conserved pathogen-associated molecular patterns, are among the receptors expressed by DCs. TLRs induce DC maturation, which regulates the activation of adaptive immune responses. It is probable that those mature DCs express self-antigens that are constantly processed and expressed about MHC class I and II molecules in addition to antigens that are absorbed at the infection site. This suggests that autoimmune T cells that have escaped thymus negative selection may become sensitized by fully competent DCs. DCs activate a number of mechanisms that may stop autoimmunity from developing in peripheral tissues. These mechanisms include peripheral autoreactive T cell deletion or anergy, antigen presentation regulation, induction/maintenance of regulatory T cells, and mechanisms that involve activation threshold tuning. One important factor in the development of immunity is the longevity of newly arrived migrant dendritics in the lymphoid organs. T cells only exhibit signs of activation 36-48 hours after forming connections with a single APC(Schneider & Sercarz, 1997). The volume and quality of $CD4^+$ T-cell responses, which are proportional to the number of antigen-carrying DCs that reach the lymph node, have been demonstrated to be significantly impacted by DC migration, which is consistent in several findings. A large number of DCs would lessen competition among T cells, promote sustained stimulation, and raise the likelihood of a DC-T cell interaction. The functioning of mature DCs in lymph nodes are not correctly identified. It has been demonstrated that splenic DCs can undergo phenotypic and functional maturation as well as fast migration in the T-cell zone upon injection of lipopolysaccharide (LPS). Very few $CD^{11}c+$ cells interact with T lymphocytes in the spleen 24 hours after the LPS injection. The LPS-induced programmed cell death in situ was significantly delayed in OVA-specific, T-cell receptor (TCR)-transgenic mice by injection of ovalbumin (OVA) peptide, indicating that T cells may rescue DCs presenting their own antigen.

2.16 Cell death

Other cell populations may initiate the programmed cell death, or it may occur naturally. The finding that growth-dependent long-term cultures of DCs exhibit three stages of maturation i.e., immature, mature, and apoptotic, supports the theory that DCs have distinct stages of life and that mature DCs die. The mature DCs survive for die earlier than immature DCs. Therefore, TLRs and T-cell costimulatory molecules activated a Bcl-xL-dependent DC survival pathway. The TLR activation subsequently caused DC apoptosis by upregulating the proapoptotic Bcl-2 family member Bim. Between days 1 and 4 of culture, the ratio of antiapoptotic to proapoptotic proteins expressed by DCs triggered by TLRs reversed due to an increase in the ratio of Bim/Bcl-2 expressed in DCs treated with LPS or lipoteichoic acid (LTA). The fact that TLR ligands establish a molecular timer indicates that mature DC apoptosis is an active process. DCs cultivated with LPS ± agonistic anti-CD40 monoclonal antibodies also experience apoptosis, indicating that T-cell signals enhance the expression of the antiapoptotic protein called Bcl-xL, which is dominated by the timer. It is yet unknown which signal or signals from the adaptive immune response could save DCs from dying too soon due to the innate system. It is believed that T-cell tolerance to self-antigens reflects both peripheral and central tolerance. Central tolerance removes autoreactive T cells by causing the thymus to delete immature T cells. The thymus-restricted production of tissue-specific antigens raises the possibility that there are other peripheral mechanisms that inhibit autoreactive T cells.

2.17 Immunogenic reactions

Not every self-protein has the ability to trigger autoimmune reactions or be immunogenic. Thyroid-stimulating hormone receptor in Graves' disease; myelin basic protein or MBP, proteolipid protein or PLP, and myelin oligodendrocyte glycoprotein or MOG in EAE/MS; H^+/K^+ ATPase in autoimmune gastritis; or insulin, glutamic acid decarboxylase (GAD), and islet-specific glucose-6-phosphatase catalytic subunit-related protein (IGRP) in T1D are among the specific self-proteins that autoreactive T-cell responses preferentially target. Even in genetic predispositions to disease, many of these antigenic T-cell specificities are tolerated, at least in part, during T-cell development. The thymocytes harboring a transgenic GAD65-reactive TCR experienced negative selection even when NOD mice mount T-cell responses to other GAD65 epitopes(Sun et al., 2023). MBP-specific T cells died of central tolerance in MBP-competent animals, but they grew properly in mice that were targeted by the MBP gene. The quantity of the relevant MHC-peptide complex on tolerogenic APCs and the target autoantigenic peptide affinity for self-MHC are both necessary for autoreactive thymocytes to be susceptible to tolerance. In MBP-competent animals, for instance, TCR-transgenic thymocytes were not destroyed by MBP1–11, which binds self-MHC with a much lower affinity than MBP121-150. Deletion was noted when the concentration or affinity of MBP1-11 (for MHC) was raised. Not all TCRs that can identify potentially tolerogenic autoantigen-MHC complexes will certainly develop tolerance; the result of T-cell development also depends on how well or poorly individual TCRs interact with particular MHC-peptide complexes. TCR-transgenic thymocytes that recognized IGRP206–214/Kd with intermediate avidity grew normally, whereas those that recognized the same complex with higher avidity did not. High-affinity autoreactive T cells may protect lower-affinity T-cells with the same antigenic specificity from tolerance induction by downregulating the corresponding MHC-peptide complex on APCs, as high-affinity T cells can remove target MHC–peptide complexes from the surface of APCs. If the target autoantigen is only expressed at low quantities of tolerogenic APCs, autoreactive T cells may avoid central tolerance(Torres-Aguilar et al., 2010).

2.18 Tolerance and other findings

Whether or not growing thymocytes come into contact with MHC-peptide complexes on medullary epithelial cells or bone marrow-derived APCs is another significant factor that determines tolerance susceptibility. Because autoreactive T cells target epitopes encoded on mRNA splice variants that are not produced in tolerogenic APCs, they can occasionally evade central tolerance. In some cases, tolerance happens even though thymic stromal cells do not express the self-antigen, as seems to be the case with IGRP206-214/Kd-reactive thymocytes. It is yet unknown if autoantigen-loaded DCs transmit IGRP206-214/Kd complexes to the thymus or if another MHC-peptide combination causes tolerance in this system. When kept in certain pathogen-free environments, transgenic mice expressing TCRs specific for multiple MBP or MOG epitopes, such as MBP1-11, MBP84-102, MBP121-150, and MOG35-55, did not develop symptoms of EAE spontaneously. However, regardless of whether the TCRs originated from encephalitogenic or non-encephalitogenic T cell clones, mice expressing PLP139-151-reactive TCRs experienced a high prevalence of disease. Similarly, in TCR-transgenic BALB/c mice, T-cells that recognized an H+/K+ ATPase α subunit epitope hardly caused autoimmune gastritis, while those that recognized an H+/K+ ATPase β subunit epitope were extremely gastritogenic(Read et al., 2007). The onset of diabetes was accelerated by the expression of the class II-restricted 4.1-TCR, but not by the expression of the BDC2.5 TCR. Compared to wild-type NOD mice, the incidence of diabetes in BDC2.5 TCR-transgenic NOD mice is much lower. When peptides generated from GAD65 were administered to young NOD mice, similar effects of antigenic specificity on pathogenicity were also noted. Certain epitopes protected the animals from T1D by stimulating Th2 cells that produce interleukin (IL)-4.

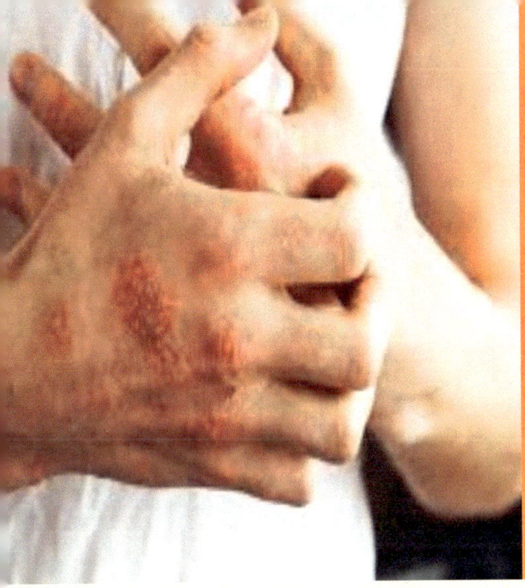

Chapter 3

APOPTOSIS AND IMMUNOGENETICS

Contents

3.1Introduction

The idea or concept that cell survival and death are strictly regulated is relatively recent, even though the appearance of cells dying by apoptosis has been known for decades. Diseases are categorized by the organ system they affect, such as the neurological, endocrine, or cardiovascular systems. Considering the mechanisms underlying the disorders is more beneficial for biomedical researchers. While many neurological diseases are brought on by the premature death of some neurons, cancers are caused by increased cell growth and survival.

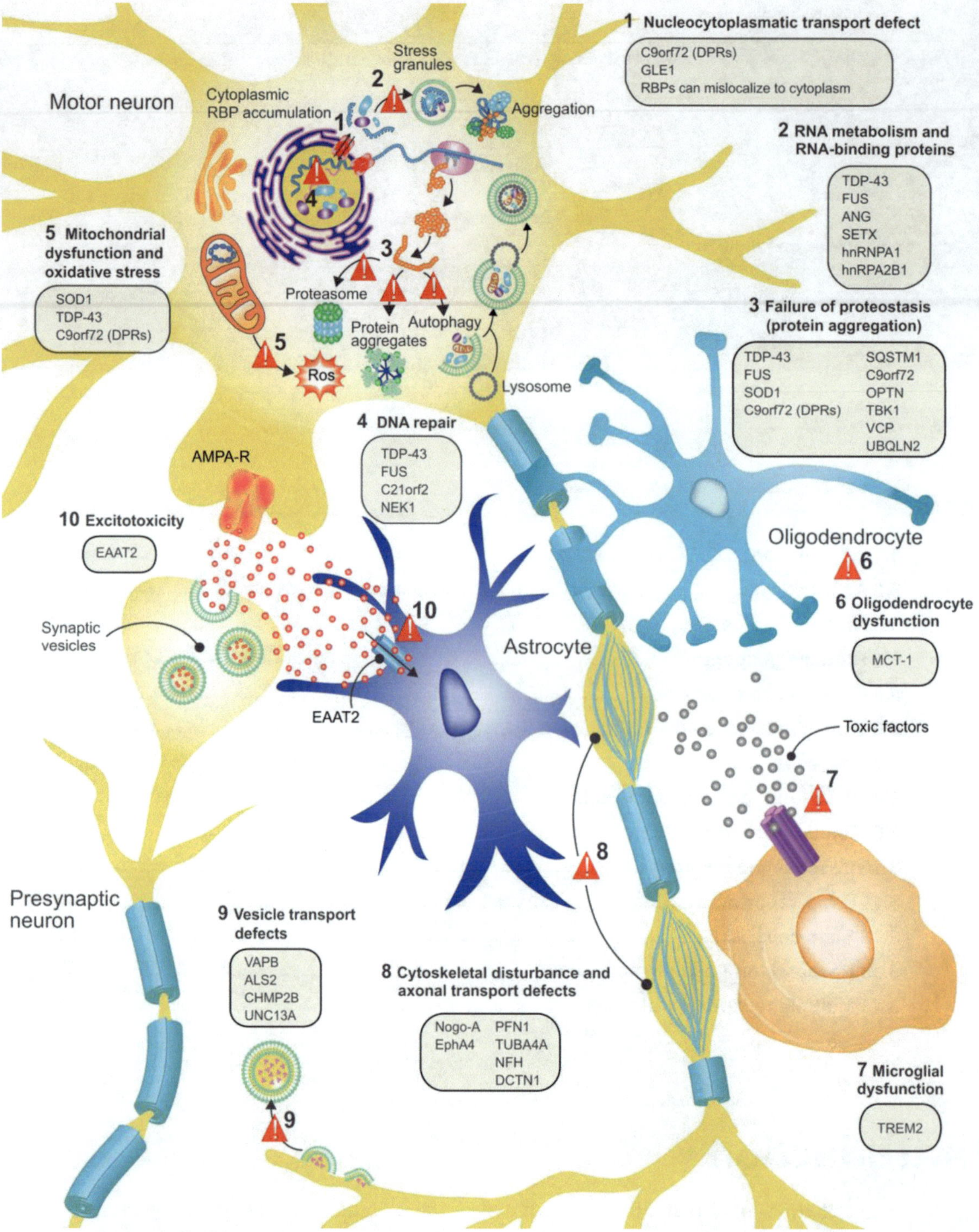

Figure 3.1 Amyotrophic lateral sclerosis

Source: https://upload.wikimedia.org/wikipedia/commons/7/76/ALS_Disease_Pathology_and_Proposed_Disease_Mechanisms.jpg,Creative Commons License.

Diseases linked to polyglutamate repeats, Alzheimer's, Parkinson's, and amyotrophic lateral sclerosis (ALS) (Figure 3.1) exhibit intracellular protein aggregates that cause apoptosis via the mitochondrial pathway(Ambegaokar et al., 2010). Since apoptosis is a crucial component of immunologic homeostasis and immunological control, aberrant cell death plays a role in the pathophysiology of these diseases. The death program consists of some essential steps like death initiation via the mitochondria, effector caspase activation, death execution via nuclease activation and cell membrane alterations, and phagocytosis. These processes are tightly controlled, and both activators and inhibitors have been found. Autoimmune disorders have complicated etiology. Environmental variables or factors control a substantial genetic component in certain disorders, such as insulin-dependent diabetes mellitus (IDDM) and systemic lupus erythematosus (SLE). Less exposure to common microbes may be linked to the rising incidence of IDDM in Western countries.

3.2 Apoptosis

The necrosis is not programmed, but apoptosis (Figure 3.2) is, and it happens through certain biochemical processes. This suggests that apoptotic death can be either triggered or stopped by pathway modulation, with therapeutic uses. Determining the mechanism of cell death in autoimmune disorders that affect certain organs is therefore crucial. Now that the criteria for differentiating between necrosis and apoptosis have been well established, it should be easy to identify which mechanism takes place in autoimmune diseases that are specific to particular organs. In many autoimmune disorders, in situ staining for DNA strand breaks (TUNEL) is nearly always positive in the affected organ; however, this test is not specific for apoptosis(Moore et al., 2021). The absence of inflammation after apoptotic cell death is a crucial difference between necrosis and apoptosis. Necrosis can be linked to the majority of autoimmune disorders.

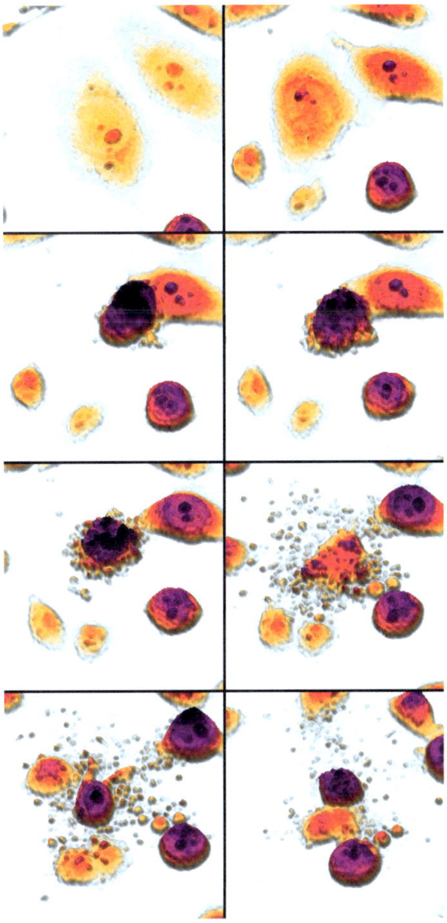

Figure 3.2 Apoptosis

Source: https://upload.wikimedia.org/wikipedia/commons/2/23/Apoptosis_DU145_cells_mosaic.jpg,*Creative Commons License.*

The fact that apoptosis or necrosis cannot be easily deduced from the type of cell present in the lesion presents another challenge in determining the form of cell death. CD8 T cells and natural killer (NK), the cell types closely linked to a death effector function, may induce cell death through the release of tumor necrosis factor (TNF)-induced necrosis or apoptosis, the perforin/granzyme pathway, or the Fas ligand

(FasL). FasL can kill CD4 T cells, but FasL expression may also operate as a chemotactic signal for neutrophils, which would most likely result in necrotic cell death if triggered. Less is known about the mechanism of cell death at the preclinical stage of human diseases, even though necrotic cell death does occur in established ailments. The pancreatic cells undergo spontaneous apoptosis. Although non-obese diabetic (NOD) and control mice appear to experience this at the same rate, pre-diabetic animals may handle apoptotic cells differently.

3.3 Autoantibodies

The long-acting thyroid stimulator (LATS) autoantibody, which functions as an agonist for the thyroid stimulating hormone (TSH) receptor on thyrocytes, is linked to Graves' disease, a kind of thyrotoxicosis(Saravanan & Dayan, 2001). It is interesting to learn that TSH inhibits the expression of Fas, which has an anti-apoptotic effect. IgG from individuals with Graves' disease mimics this action. Other researchers, however, have not been able to verify alterations in Fas expression when thyrocytes were exposed to TSH in vitro. In contrast to T cells in Hashimoto's disease, which express Th1 cytokines, T cells in Graves' disease produce Th2 cytokines. The two completely different diseases result from the actions of cytokines: Th2 cytokines increase Fas resistance by promoting the expression of c-FLIP and Bcl-XL (Graves' disease), while IFN-γ increases susceptibility to Fas-mediated apoptosis (Hashimoto's thyroiditis). Scleroderma and RA are two rheumatic diseases linked to fibroblast activation and proliferation, although the underlying mechanisms are not well known. The cytokine strongly linked to the fibrosis and skin thickening seen in scleroderma is transforming growth factor (TGF)-β. Determining how a cytokine like TGF-β may be linked to the development of cells like fibroblasts but to cell cycle arrest and/or lymphocyte death is crucial. The development of tissue known as the pannus that infiltrates bone and cartilage is a characteristic of RA. Several cytokines and growth factors (GF) contribute to the formation of the pannus, but the therapeutic efficacy of TNF- α blockade indicates that TNF-α is an essential part of this pathological process. In the majority of cells, TNF-α activates NF-kB, which in turn triggers a series of anti-apoptotic and inflammatory mediators. NF-B may interfere with GADD45 and inhibit apoptosis by blocking the janus kinase (JNK) pathway(Zerbini & Libermann, 2005). Understanding how the signal transduction pathways differ would have a significant impact on treatments for inflammatory diseases because TNF-α may also cause cell death.

Programmed cell death, or apoptosis, is a term that, unlike necrosis, suggests that a dying cell actively participates in its own death. Many internal and external signals have the ability to start this process. Apoptosis helps developing vertebrates and invertebrates control the number of cells and the production of tissues. Mature organisms continue this physiological program, which aims to preserve steady cellular homeostasis. However, there is evidence that apoptosis, or cell death, also contributes to many disease conditions. It is believed that apoptotic cell death plays a role in mediating tissue and organ damage brought on by environmental stresses like hypoxia, trauma, and infection. While excessive apoptosis is thought to play a role in the pathophysiology of certain chronic degenerative disorders, insufficient apoptosis has been connected to diseases like cancer. The significance of apoptosis in the immune system is supported by the finding that dysregulated apoptosis can result in several ailments, such as autoimmune diseases, lymphoid malignancies, or immunological suppression brought on by excessive lymphocyte death. Programmed cell death is crucial for many stages of T and B cell development and subsequent functional life. By removing lymphocytes that do not express an antigen receptor, apoptosis aids in the early establishment of a functional repertoire of mature cells. Expansion and differentiation depend on the expression of both cytokine receptors and the pre-T cell receptor (TCR); if survival signals are not supplied through both receptors, CD4 - CD8 cells experience apoptosis(Haks et al., 1999). Apoptosis is also how T cells are eliminated during the later stages of development, which include positive and negative selection. In the MHC molecules, CD4/CD8 double-positive thymocytes that express TCR with a reasonable affinity for peptide ligands undergo differentiation into either CD4 or CD8 single-positive cells during this stage. However, T cells that express TCR with poor peptide affinity are neglected and die as a result of not receiving enough survival impulses. The clonal elimination of these potentially autoreactive cells results from an excessively high-affinity TCR interaction with self-MHC. Apoptosis in the bone marrow destroys B cells that can identify self-antigens. Therefore, apoptosis plays a crucial role in lymphocyte development by ensuring the removal of both non-functional and autoreactive cells.

Another essential element of the developed immune system is programmed cell death. A component of the adaptive immune response is the clonal proliferation of antigen-specific cells. To prevent negative consequences like an autoimmune reaction or possible cancer, it is crucial to effectively eliminate these activated, proliferating cells once an infection has been effectively eliminated. By eliminating activated cells, apoptosis serves to preserve homeostasis in this scenario. The lymphocytes die due to a shortage of trophic substances, or by activation-induced cell death (AICD), a process that induces apoptosis through repeated TCR stimulation. Similarly, B cell receptor (BCR) activation can cause activated B cells to undergo apoptosis. Researchers have made good progress in understanding the mechanisms of apoptosis.

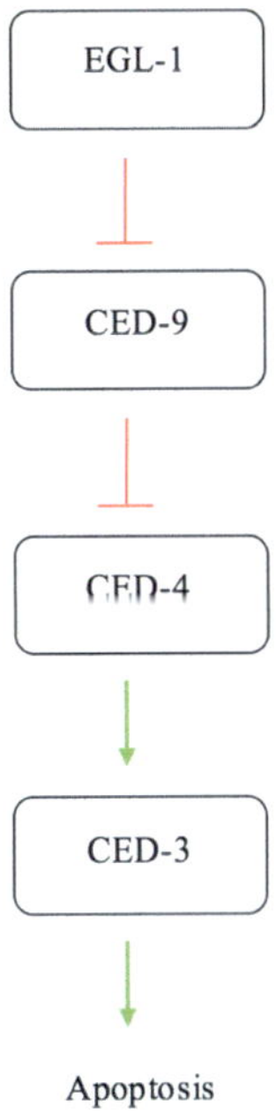

Figure 3.3 Apoptosis in *Caenorhabditis elegans*

Source: By DanaMarie217 - Own work, CC BY-SA 4.0, https://commons.wikimedia.org/w/index.php?curid=64477110,*Creative Commons License.*

The research of animals lacking some caspases like cysteinyl aspartate proteases and other associated proteins has contributed to our understanding of the complexities of apoptosis. Studies of their homologs in *Caenorhabditis elegans*(Figure 3.3) led to the initial recognition of the critical role that caspases play in cell death. Loss-of-function mutations of the proteins CED-3 and CED-4 were first found in *C.elegans*with deficient apoptosis, indicating their importance for apoptosis(Horowitz & Shaham, 2024). The protein CED-9 has since been discovered to be an apoptosis inhibitor that acts upstream of CED-3 and CED-4. Loss-of-function CED-3 or CED-4 mutations can reverse the phenotype of embryonic mortality caused by increased apoptosis caused by loss-of-function CED-9 mutations. Apoptosis is also suppressed by loss-of-function mutations of the protein EGL-1, which interacts with CED-9(Liu & Hengartner, 1999). CED-9 functions as a negative regulator of apoptosis by binding to and inhibiting CED-4.

3.4 Proteins in apoptosis

These proteins were analyzed, and it was shown that CED-3 is a caspase that is similar to the mammalian interleukin (IL)-1-converting enzyme (ICE or caspase-1). The discovery that CED-3 is essential for apoptosis led to the search for additional mammalian caspases that might have a comparable function. There are 14 human caspases, and the resulting pathways are more complex as a result, even though the overall apoptotic system that has evolved for higher animals is preserved from *C.elegans*. Mammalian counterparts of the caspases and the other components of the *C.elegans* apoptotic process have also been discovered. Apoptosis can be distinguished from necrotic cell death by a variety of alterations in cellular morphology, although there are no standards for defining it. Chromosomes shrink, the nucleus breaks apart, the cytoplasmic volume drops, organelles condense, the cell membrane joins the endoplasmic reticulum, and the cell ultimately breaks up into several apoptotic bodies, which are then consumed by neighboring cells. Other intracellular markers of apoptosis, such as a drop in mitochondrial transmembrane potential and the exposure of phosphatidylserine on the cell membrane exterior, accompany these morphologic changes. One significant feature of this unique cellular packaging is that apoptosis does not include the inflammation and potential harm to neighboring cells that necrosis does. At least some of the subcellular alterations that occur during apoptosis are caused by caspases cleaving specific subcellular proteins. Of all the proteases, caspases have one of the substrate specificities; they always cleave aspartate residues on the carboxyl side. The peptide motif QACXG has a conserved cysteine residue that, in conjunction with conserved glycine and histidine, contributes to the catalytic site(Chou et al., 2000).

3.5 Catalysis and domains

Cells include inactive monomeric zymogens called caspases, which are made up of a large subunit, a small subunit, and an N-terminal prodomain. Processing takes place in locations (sites) between the domains that have aspartate residues, which is compatible with the capacity of procaspase to autoactivate or be triggered by other caspases. The functioning heterotetrameric enzyme, a complex of two large and two tiny subunits with two distinct active sites, is formed when two zymogen precursors are cleaved at these locations, releasing the subunits. It has been discovered that the long prodomains contain either caspase recruitment domains (CARD) or death effector domains (DED), which can interact with adaptor molecules and cause pro-caspases to cluster. The zymogen low, intrinsic autocatalytic activity may be enhanced by this close contact, enabling it to cleave and activate itself. The adaptor molecule FADD or Fas-associated death domain protein or Mort-1 is recruited by oligomerization of the Fas receptor via their death domains (DD). The death-inducing signaling complex (DISC) can be recruited by a DED on pro-caspase-8 through interaction with the DED on the other end of FADD. This induced proximity allows pro-caspase-8 to activate itself after it has been recruited. It is also believed that Caspase-10, which has a DED, interacts with FADD. The connections between pro-caspase-2 and RAIDD/CRADD and pro-caspase-9 and Apaf-1 are known to be mediated by CARD(Reed, 2000). Once triggered, caspases with long prodomains or initiators are believed to cleave caspases with short domains, known as effectors, which then execute the apoptotic program. For instance, there is proof that caspase-3 can cleave caspase-8 and -9 upstream, and it may possibly have the ability to autoactivate. Human caspase-4 is similar to mouse caspase-11. In HeLa and Rat-1 cells, overexpression of caspase-11 triggers apoptosis, which Bcl-2 and CrmA can prevent. Because LPS strongly induces caspase-11 expression, it may play a regulatory function in both inflammatory reactions and apoptosis. Although caspase-11 does not directly process pro-IL-1, caspase-1 processes pro-IL-1 when caspase-11 is overexpressed.

Analysis of knockout mice demonstrated how important caspase-1 is for acute inflammatory reactions. Mice lacking caspase-1 exhibit better survival and reduced production of IL-1, IL-6, and tumor necrosis factor (TNF)-α, in addition to being less susceptible to the effects of lipopolysaccharide (LPS)-induced shock than their wild-type counterparts (animals). It is interesting to observe that mice lacking caspase-11 exhibit a comparable survival benefit in shock caused by LPS. The findings that caspase-11 is absolutely necessary for caspase-1 activity and that the two molecules are found in the same protein complex within cells point to a mechanism in which the two molecules must interact in order for activity and cytokine processing to occur.

3.6 Transgenic cell studied

It has been demonstrated that CD^{30} knockout results in a partial deficiency in eliminating self-reactive transgenic $CD8^+$ T cells in male mice utilizing H-Y transgenic mice, in which the TCR detects a Y chromosomal antigen, leading to clonal deletion by negative selection in the male thymus. TCR and CD30 crosslinking reagents increase programmed cell death in the mouse thymus when CD30 is overexpressed. In this case, CD30 activates caspase-1, which could cause negative selection. However, research indicates that CD30-deficient animals can perform negative selection of both anti-self $CD4^+$ and $CD8^+$ T cells, raising uncertainties about the crucial role of CD30 in negative selection. However, more research on this aspect of negative selection is necessary. One possible approach is to create TCR transgenic mice that recognize endogenous antigen, such as a peptide presented by MHC, and track the deletion of T cells in these mice using caspase-$1^{-/-}$ or -$11^{-/-}$ backgrounds. Since these mice have not been shown to develop systemic autoimmune diseases, their potential contribution to peripheral tolerance is probably minimal. Pro-caspase-8 is then activated and released from the DISC into the cytoplasm as a result of proteolytic cleavage, which is likely an autocatalyzed event aided by the proximity of several caspase-8 zymogens recruited to the death-inducing signaling complex or DISC. There are two methods in which the caspase-8 downstream signal spreads, depending on the cell environment. When apoptosis is induced in type I cells, the DESC activates a significant amount of caspase-8. Following the quick cleavage and activation of caspase-3 by caspase-8, apoptosis enters the effector stage. However, in type II cells, the loss of mitochondrial transmembrane potential leads to a significant decrease in DISC formation and the activation of caspase-8 and -3(Keresztes & Streicher, 2017).

3.7 Caspases

The pro-apoptotic Bcl-2 family member Bid is cleaved and activated by caspase-8 in this caspase cascade variation(Fischer et al., 2003). Truncated Bid causes mitochondrial pore formation through Bak or Bax, which releases pro-apoptotic chemicals such as cytochrome c and Smac/DIABLO. After that, cytochrome c can combine with Apaf-1 and pro-caspase-9 in the cytoplasm to create the apoptosome, which can subsequently trigger effector caspases like caspase-3 and -7. Apoptosis in type I cells does not require mitochondrial activation, even though it can happen in type II cells as well. Although it is not as essential as its counterpart CED-3, which is necessary for programmed cell death (*C. elegans*), caspase-3 has established itself as a central regulator caspase in mammals. The variety of possible caspase-3 substrates and the confluence of the death-receptor and mitochondrial-mediated death pathways at caspase-3 activation support this function of caspase-3. Although caspase-3 is crucial for the development of neurons, it appears to be optional for the growing lymphoid system because animals lacking caspase-3 exhibit normal T and B cell development. Without caspase-3, thymocyte apoptosis brought on by anti-CD3 crosslinking or anti-Fas remains unchanged, indicating that caspase-2 does not influence at least some component of negative selection. In the absence of an important caspase, mammalian cells can trigger apoptosis through compensatory caspase activation.

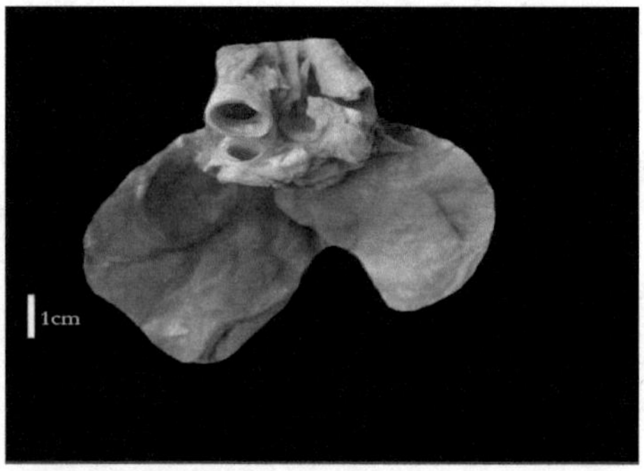

Figure 3.4 Thymus

Source: https://upload.wikimedia.org/wikipedia/commons/1/11/Human_thymus_posterior_view.jpg,*Creative Commons License.*

In the thymus, (Figure 3.4) death (apoptosis) during T-cell growth has been demonstrated to be mediated by both p53 and Bcl-2. T-cell development seems to be normal in mice lacking caspase-3. Research studies employing some methods that inhibit all thymus caspase activity were unable to identify a deficit in this kind of cell death. According to some findings, death by neglect in T cell development may necessitate a mechanism that depends on p53 and Bcl-2 rather than caspases. Following infection, T cells are stimulated to expand clonally by antigen-presenting cells, specifically dendritic cells, which deliver antigenic peptides of the infectious pathogens. The number of antigen-reactive lymphocytes must decrease until the pool of lymphoid cells approaches a baseline level following a phase of clonal expansion. Activation-induced cell death or AICD accomplishes this by balancing apoptosis, which typically happens through death receptors characterized by Fas, with growth/expansion. AICD is lacking in activated T cells from caspase-3-/-mice. When compared to wild-type controls, caspase-3$^{-/-}$ peripheral T cells demonstrated decreased cell death following exposure to superantigen staphylococcal enterotoxin A (SEA). Anti-CD3 or anti-Fas antibodies enhance the viability of activated caspase-3$^{-/-}$ lymphocytes. These findings suggest that caspase-3 is necessary for peripheral T-cell AICD. Systemic autoimmune diseases like lupus have been directly associated with deficiencies in the Fas signaling pathway. The impact of caspase deficiency in this type of autoimmune disease should be the main focus of future research. The death of peripheral T and B cells can occur in many ways besides AICD. High levels of TCR signaling, the removal of growth factors like IL-2 or IL-15 from T cells, or the lack of a tonic TCR signal on naïve T cells can cause peripheral T cell death(Boyman et al., 2012).

After it was observed that adding ATP or dATP to cell extracts made from normally developing cells starts an apoptotic program as indicated by caspase-3 activation and DNA fragmentation, the caspase-9 activation route was identified. Recent biochemical research discovered a protein complex made up of cytochrome c and Apaf-1 that may attract and activate pro-caspase-9 when ATP or dATP is hydrolyzed. Pro-caspase-9 catalytic activity is not considerably increased by proteolytic processing, even though caspases are typically activated by cleavage. Instead, caspase-9 interaction with its protein cofactors, cytochrome c, and Apaf-1, is essential for its activation. When combined, they create the active holoenzyme, also known as the apoptosome.

Mice lacking either apoptotic protease activating factor 1 (Apaf-1) or caspase-9 have been used to demonstrate the importance of the apoptosome in vivo. The caspase-3 activation is eliminated in the developing brain of caspase-9$^{-/-}$ embryos and these abnormalities are similar to those of caspase-3$^{-/-}$ mice. The cytochrome c deletion demonstrates the apoptosome function in programmed cell death. Although a study of knockout embryo-derived cell lines shows resilience to apoptosis produced by ultraviolet (UV) irradiation, serum withdrawal, and staurosporine, these animals die prenatally, likely as a result of the failure in aerobic metabolism. However, it is interesting to note that cytochrome c $^{-/-}$ cells seem to be more susceptible to TNF-α induced mortality. These mice T cell development was normal, in contrast to the impact of caspase-9 and Apaf-1 loss on neural development. Both Apaf-1$^{-/-}$ and caspase-9$^{-/-}$ thymocytes exhibit resistance to apoptosis when exposed to stimuli like dexamethasone and radiation. The thymocytes of the wild type, Apaf-1$^{-/-}$, and caspase-9-/- are susceptible to Fas-mediated apoptosis, indicating that Fas-mediated cell death in thymocytes occurs independently of the Apaf1/caspase-9 pathway. The absence of abnormalities in T cell development further implies that Apaf-1 and caspase-9 are not involved in thymus death or damage.

3.8 Mitochondria and apoptosis

Recent research has demonstrated that a positive feedback loop mediated by mitochondria plays a role in the tumor-induced death of activated T cells. These results show that cleavage of Bid is one of the steps that follow the loss of mitochondrial transmembrane potential, which appears to be independent of death receptor signaling. This further increases mitochondrial permeability and triggers apoptosome activation. Even though it has been shown that these mutations do not affect Fas-mediated thymocyte death, it is crucial to investigate whether the Apaf-1/caspase-9 pathway plays a role in the death of activated T cells. Mutations in Apaf-1 and caspase-9 can also prevent p53-induced cell death in embryonic fibroblasts that express c-Myc and Ras(McCarthy et al., 2001). By activating Apaf1 and caspase-9, p53 may influence negative selection. Although p53 deficiency partially restores development to CD4^{+}CD8^{+} pre-T cells in SCID, Rag1$^{-/-}$, and Rag2$^{-/-}$ mice, it may also mediate death by neglect at the pre-TCR stage. Thymus hyperplasia and thymoma are caused by p53 or pro-apoptotic Bcl-2 family members losing their activity. The Bcl-2 family, whose members regulate the mitochondrial-directed activation of Apaf1 and caspase-9, has also been studied concerning the molecular mechanisms driving apoptosis in the immune system. Early postnatal death is caused by a deficiency of the anti-apoptotic Bcl-2 protein, but lymphocyte growth is initially normal. Bcl-x deficient mice, on the other hand, are embryonic lethal due to severe neuronal apoptosis and decreased survival of immature lymphocytes. These mice lack both the pro-apoptotic Bcl-xS and the anti-apoptotic Bcl-xL. CD4^{+}CD8^{+} thymocyte survival was decreased in Rag2$^{-/-}$ mice chimeras containing Bcl-x$^{-/-}$ embryonic stem cells, but adult single-positive cell survival remained unaffected(Li et al., 2010). A deficiency in the proapoptotic Bcl-2 family member Bim led to a rise in mature single-positive and CD4-CD8- lymphocytes, but interestingly, a decrease in $CD4^{+}CD8^{+}$ cells. Bim-deficient animals also showed an age-dependent autoimmune disease, peripheral lymphoid organ hyperplasia, and elevated leukocyte counts.

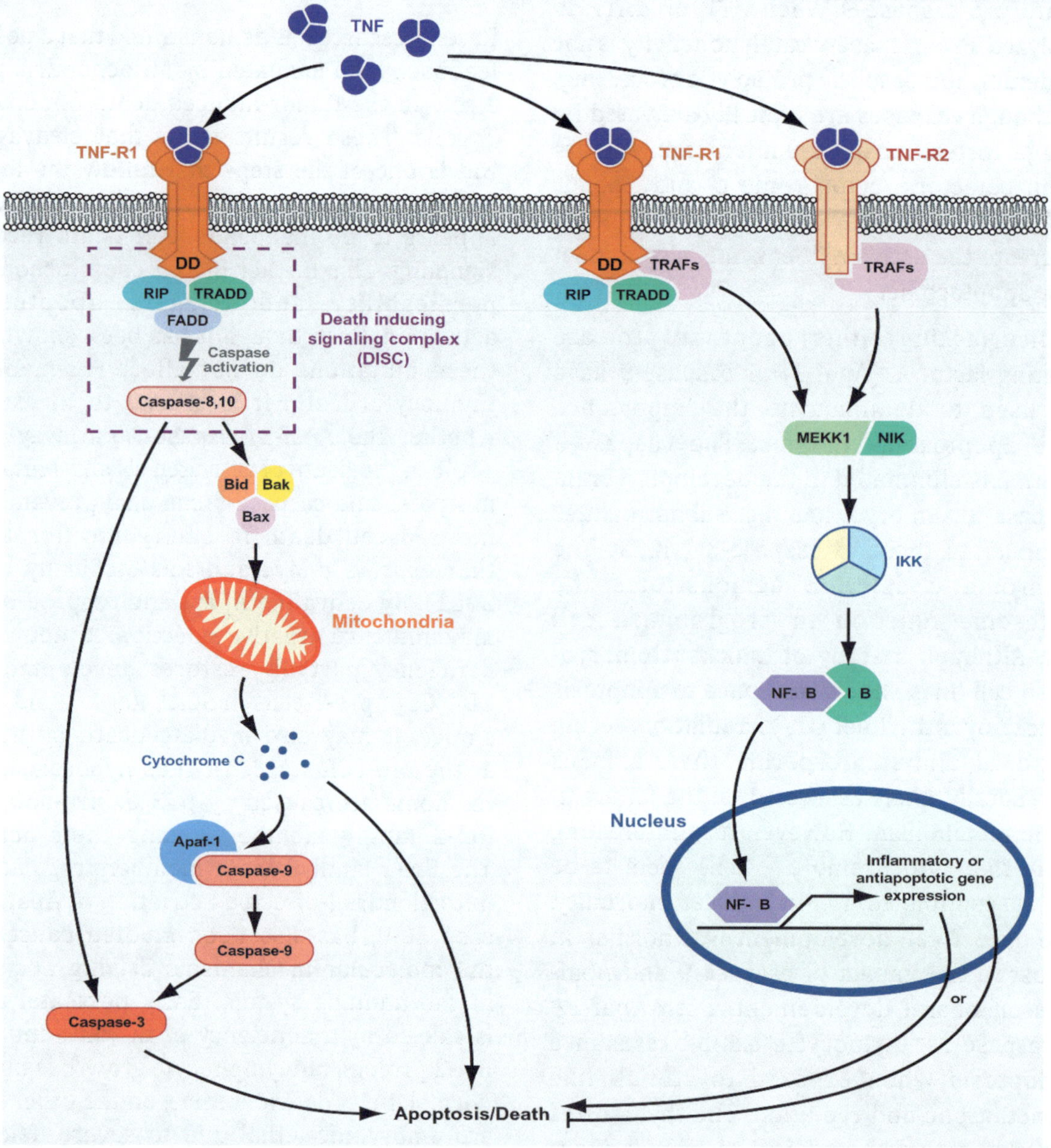

Figure 3.5 TNF-mediated apoptosis

Source: https://upload.wikimedia.org/wikipedia/commons/c/c6/TNF-Mediated_Death_and_Survival_Pathways.png,*Creative Commons License.*

This suggests that there may be a mitochondrial-mediated death pathway that is not dependent on caspase-9 and that counteracts caspase-9 deficit by compensatory activation of other caspases, such as caspase-2. Initially discovered to be a type of mRNA that was strongly expressed in the developing mouse brain, caspase-2 was later found to be down-regulated in the adult mouse. Because of its long prodomain, which suggests an upstream initiator role, caspase-2 location in apoptotic pathways is difficult to understand. Although the biological importance of this interaction is still unknown, its prodomain caspase-recruitment domain (CARD) enables it to engage with the adaptor protein CRADD/RAIDD effectively. Because caspase and receptor interacting protein (RIP) adaptor with death domain (CRADD)/ RIP-associated ICH-1/CED-3 homologous protein with a death domain (RAIDD) has a DD, it can interact with receptor interacting protein (RIP), an enzyme that connects to the TNF-RI through the adaptor molecule TRADD. RAIDD/caspase-2 interactions are not necessary, at least not in this cell type, as Caspase-2-deficient embryonic fibroblasts are susceptible to TNF-mediated apoptosis (Figure 3.5).

3.9 Mutation-based studies

The data from cell-free extracts stimulated with cytochrome c suggests that caspase-3 can activate caspase-2 in a manner that is dependent on caspase-9, suggesting that it may function as a downstream effector as opposed to an upstream initiator. The predominant type, caspase-2L, promotes apoptosis. However, caspase-2S, a condensed product produced by inserting an early stop codon, has anti-apoptotic properties. The deletion of caspase-2 in mice is the sole instance of a caspase knockout with evidence of both pro- and anti-apoptotic effects. The caspase-2L variant is expressed by mouse ovarian germ cells. These germ cells in the caspase-2 mutant animals were immune to doxorubicin exposure during ovarian development, which typically results in the death of half to two-thirds of germ cells(Lakhani et al., 2002).

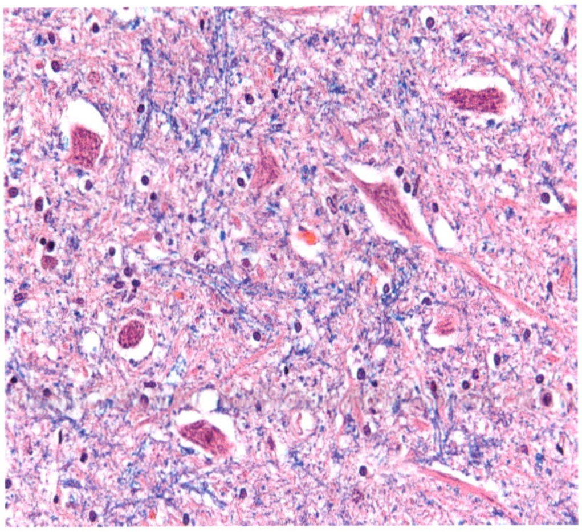

Figure 3.6 Facial motor neurons

Source: https://upload.wikimedia.org/wikipedia/commons/8/8f/Medulla_oblongata_-_posterior_-_cn_xii_-_very_high_mag.jpg,*Creative Commons License.*

The mutant animals displayed fewer cells during late embryogenesis in facial motor neurons, (Figure 3.6) where both caspase-2L and -2S are believed to be expressed, suggesting an increase in apoptosis. However, the deletion has the same number of cells as the wild-type by postnatal day 7, suggesting that apoptosis has decreased. It was discovered that in response to growth factor withdrawal, caspase-$2^{-/-}$ sympathetic neurons underwent apoptosis more successfully than wild-type neurons. It appears from these findings that caspase-2 actions vary depending on the specific tissue and developmental stage. It has also been demonstrated that caspase-2 is essential for neuronal apoptosis brought on by amyloid, a protein that builds up in Alzheimer's patient brains and is thought to play a part in the pathogenesis of the condition. Sympathetic neurons from caspase-2 mutant animals are resistant to amyloid-induced apoptosis.

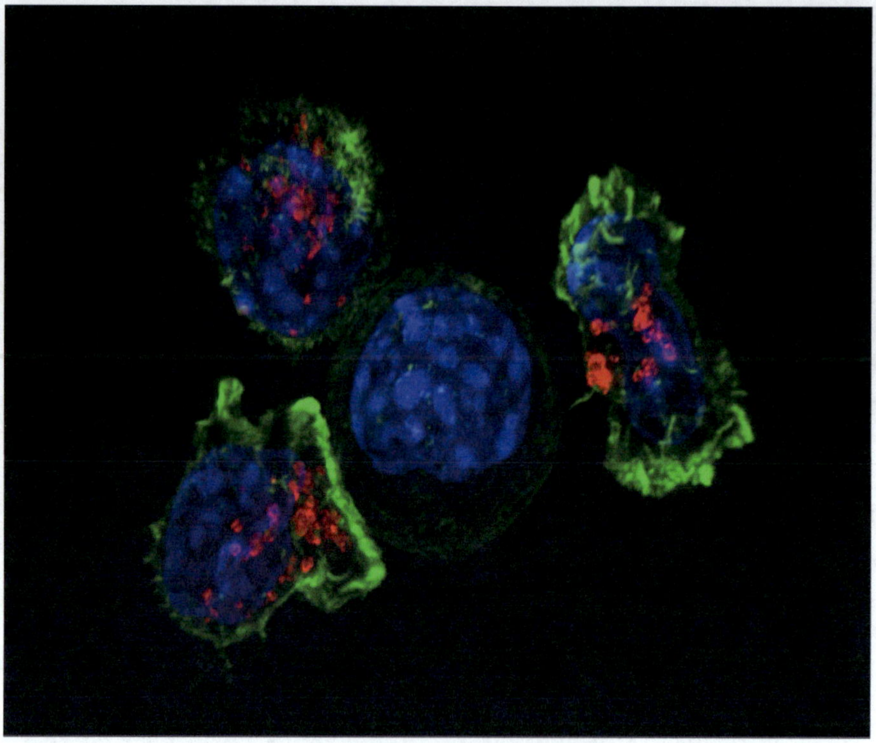

Figure 3.7 Cytotoxic T lymphocytes

Source: https://upload.wikimedia.org/wikipedia/commons/a/aa/Killer_T_cells_surround_a_cancer_cell.png,*Creative Commons License.*

The cytotoxic T lymphocytes (CTL) (Figure 3.7) can cause apoptosis in target cells by releasing the serine protease granzyme B and perforin, which was used to assess lymphocyte death in caspase-2 mutant mice(Edwards et al., 1999). B lymphoblasts from caspase-2 mutant mice were resistant to apoptosis produced by granzyme B/perforin, but not to anti-Fas, doxorubicin, or staurosporine, which is consistent with the capacity of granzyme B to cleave caspase-2 in vitro. These animals have not yet been shown to exhibit symptoms of autoimmune disease, even though CTL-mediated apoptosis is thought to be a crucial mechanism for eliminating activated B cells after an immune response. The endoplasmic reticulum or ER, an organelle involved in protein synthesis, folding, and trafficking, is susceptible to changes in protein homeostasis. When this system is disturbed, for example, by the buildup of misfolded proteins or by many other ER effects, such as oxidative stress, glycosylation inhibitors, or calcium ionophores, the ER stress response is triggered, which can ultimately result in apoptosis. The discovery that caspase-12 (Figure 3.8) localizes to the ER suggests that it may be involved in the ER stress response. Mice without Caspase-12 exhibit no discernible developmental defects and are alive. Similar to how knockout embryonic fibroblasts are typically susceptible to apoptosis from anti-Fas, TNF-α, and staurosporine, knockout thymocytes were typically susceptible to apoptosis produced by anti-Fas and dexamethasone. But when exposed to ER stressors such as tunicamycin, and brefeldin A, embryonic fibroblasts with caspase-12$^{-/-}$ demonstrated resistance to apoptosis.

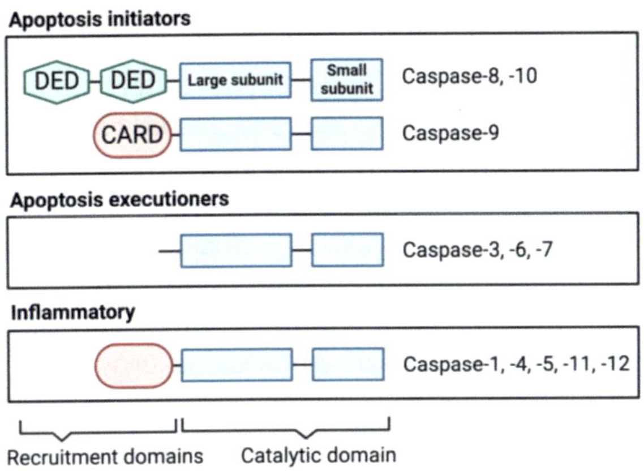

Figure 3.8 Caspases

Source: Bibo-Verdugo, Betsaida, and Guy Salvesen. 2024. "Evolution of Caspases and the Invention of Pyroptosis" International Journal of Molecular Sciences 25, no. 10: 5270. https://doi.org/10.3390/ijms25105270,*Creative Commons License.*

It was demonstrated that mutant mice had less apoptosis and damage to renal tubular cells using an in vivo model of tunicamycin-mediated renal epithelial cell death. It is interesting to note that primary cortical neurons from animals lacking caspase-12 do not die when exposed to β-amyloid, suggesting that β-amyloid works, at least in part, by creating ER stress. However, it is still unknown how ER stress leads to caspase-12 activation. However, there is evidence that the protease calpain is activated by the release of calcium (intracellular) reserves linked to ER stress, which can then activate caspase-12 and cause apoptosis. The capacity of related proteins to compensate for the loss of function has made it challenging to evaluate the contributions of individual proteins, even though the creation of knockout mice has expanded our understanding of the cellular apoptotic machinery. This has been demonstrated in several scenarios, including a model of Fas-mediated cell death in hepatocytes, which are type II cells that carry out apoptosis through the mitochondrial pathway. The activation of alternative caspases in hepatocytes from caspase-9 or caspase-3 knockout animals could still result in cell death from anti-Fas antibody, however, the patterns of caspase activation differed between wild-type and knockouts. Hepatocytes with caspase-$3^{-/-}$ demonstrated activation of caspase-6 and -7, which is not observed in the wild-type, and hepatocytes with caspase-$9^{-/-}$ demonstrated activation of caspase-2 and -6, which is likewise not observed in the wild-type. A double Bax/Bak knockout results in a severe phenotype that includes perinatal lethality, persistence of interdigital webbing, CNS or central nervous system hyperplasia, splenomegaly, and resistance to Fas-induced hepatocyte apoptosis, in contrast to a single knockout of either Bax or Bak, which produces viable mice with only mild apoptotic defects.

3.10 Caspase modifications

Strain-specific caspase activity-modifying variables are probably present and could influence how the data are interpreted. These findings support the idea that if a caspase function can be performed by another caspase, it is challenging to rule it out as important for a cell death pattern. To further understand apoptotic pathways, we will need to keep researching knockout combinations. It is also critical to understand that pharmacotherapeutic strategies for diseases that target caspase pathways would require inhibiting many caspases to get the intended result. There is evidence that caspases other than caspase-1 and -11 can have additional functions in the immune system, although caspase research has mostly focused on their roles in apoptosis. TCR stimulation activates caspase-8 but not caspase-9. The caspase activity leads to a selective cleavage of the substrate because it processes poly(ADP-ribose) polymerase or

PARP, but not replication factor C or RFC140 or DNA fragmentation factor or DFF45(Chang & Yang, 2000). Anti-CD3-induced human T cell proliferation and IL-2 production are inhibited by caspase activity inhibitors. Therefore, caspase activation seems to be involved in the initial stages of lymphocyte activation and may constitute an early physiological response in live, stimulated cells. Death receptors like Fas, TNF-related apoptosis-inducing ligand (TRAIL), and TNF-R are stimulated to activate caspase during TCR triggering. The fact that Fas activation can cause cell proliferation in certain experimental systems lends credibility to this idea. Recent research has demonstrated that the proto-oncogene c-fos, a target gene of mitogenic stimuli, is up-regulated when Jurkat T cells are stimulated with FasL or the closely related TRAIL. It was demonstrated that T cell activation is influenced by Fas-associated death domain (FADD), a molecule upstream of initiator caspases. In addition to being resistant to FasL-mediated apoptosis, T cells lacking FADD or expressing a dominant-negative mutant allele of FADD could not also proliferate in response to TCR stimulation.

3.11 Other reports

Red blood cell synthesis is the result of the successive development of proerythroblasts and basophilic or immature erythroblasts, polychromatophilic and orthochromatic, and enucleated red cells from erythroid progenitors. Several death receptors are expressed by immature erythroid cells, and adult erythroblasts produce their ligands. When erythroid progenitors were exposed to adult erythroblasts or death-receptor ligands, the transcription factor GATA-1 was degraded by caspase, which is linked to poor erythroblast development. Activation of the death receptor triggers the impact of differentiation arrest, which occurs independently of cell death. Thus, the cleavage of GATA-1 by caspase may be a crucial negative regulatory mechanism that regulates the differentiation of immature erythroblasts into mature erythroblasts. The differentiation of adult erythroblasts into enucleated red blood cells also involves caspase activation. During terminal erythroid differentiation, erythroblast morphology undergoes significant alterations, including enucleation, organelle loss, and chromatin condensation. Certain morphological alterations that result from caspase activation during apoptosis have characteristics in common. Early in the differentiation process, before the nucleus and chromatin condensation, caspase inhibitors stop the maturation of human erythroid progenitors. During erythroblast development, effector caspases like caspase-3 are activated via the mitochondrial pathway. They cleave proteins involved in chromatin condensation (acinus) and nucleus integrity (lamin B) without causing cell death or GATA-1 cleavage(Ribeil et al., 2007). Thus, for erythroblasts to undergo terminal differentiation, caspase activation and substrate selection are essential. Caspases seem to work during differentiating through at least two related mechanisms: either they can deplete particular proteins to rearrange the internal structure of the cell or they can cleave transcription factors that program the cell fate. Other cell types probably employ these same processes, particularly when lymphocytes are differentiating. Depending on their substrates, caspases may play a role in both the death of blast T cells and the process of terminal differentiation to memory cells during memory T cell production. Another example is SATB1, a transcription factor that is processed by caspase-6 in activated T cells and has been demonstrated to be essential for T and B cell differentiation. It would be interesting to see whether this behavior persists in mice lacking caspase-6 in vivo.

Damaged or excess cells must be removed quickly, and without causing organ damage or inflammation to preserve an organism ability to operate. Cellular death, also known as apoptosis, can be activated by extrinsic stimuli at a specific developmental stage. An evolutionarily conserved cell death program is triggered by different stimuli and signaling pathways, leading to changes in the cell membrane, the cleavage of many proteins by caspase, and the cleavage of nuclear DNA by DNase. In contrast to necrotic cell death, apoptotic cell death is characterized by the lack of tissue damage and an inflammatory response.

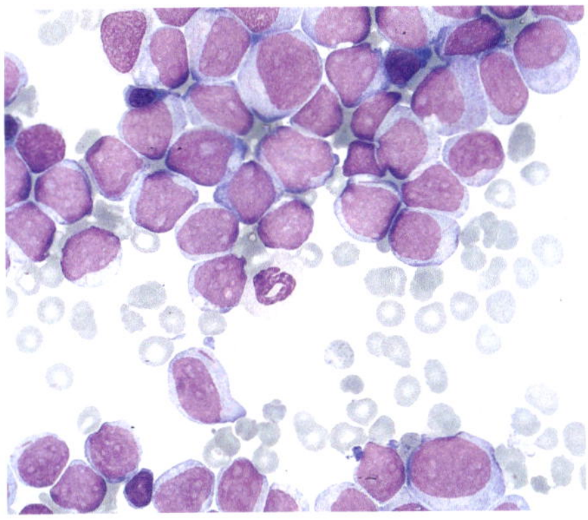

Figure 3.9 Myeloid stem cells

Source: https://upload.wikimedia.org/wikipedia/commons/2/21/Acute_Myeloid_Leukemia_%28M2_type%29.jpg,*Creative Commons License.*

The fact that apoptotic cells preserve their membrane integrity and contain phagocyte recognition signals, which target apoptotic cells for phagocytosis before cell lysis, was frequently cited as the explanation for the lack of inflammation at locations of enhanced apoptosis. As a result, harmful substances like proteolytic enzymes that may cause tissue damage and inflammation are not expelled from apoptotic cells. It has been noted that once apoptotic cells are engulfed, pro-inflammatory mediators such thromboxane B2, which are typically produced in macrophages upon phagocytosis, are not released. Although it is yet unknown why various apoptotic cell death inducers, such as ultraviolet (UV) light and X-rays, effectively reduce a variety of inflammatory disorders, these pathways may account for the lack of inflammation and tissue damage at apoptotic sites. According to recent findings, apoptotic cells actually cause monocytes and macrophages to produce anti-inflammatory and immunosuppressive cytokines while inhibiting the production of pro-inflammatory cytokines.

3.12 Stem cells

Myeloid stem cells (Figure 3.9) in the bone marrow give rise to monocytes. The majority of monocytes escape into the tissues and develop into macrophages after a short circulation in the peripheral blood. Although numerous subsets of monocytes and macrophages have been identified based on their phenotype and function, the physiological roles of these subsets remain unclear. Together with polymorphonuclear leukocytes, monocytes and macrophages are the primary phagocytic cells. Due to their ability to phagocytose, digest, and present pathogen-derived peptides to T helper cells in the form of major histocompatibility complex class II (MHC II) molecules, they are crucial antigen-presenting cells (APCs)(Sant, 2019). Activated macrophages contribute significantly to the activation of memory T lymphocytes because they express MHC II in addition to co-stimulatory molecules like B7-1/B7-2. Macrophages are unable to effectively activate naïve T lymphocytes, unlike DCs. Although many cells, such as fibroblasts and endothelial cells, take part in the uptake of dead adjacent cells, macrophages may be the most effective feeders of apoptotic cells. Through macropinocytosis, apoptotic cells are engulfed, most likely through a mechanism involving several receptors. We need to examine the cytokine secretion patterns of pure monocytes and peripheral blood mononuclear cells (PBMCs) in the presence and absence of apoptotic cells to determine whether these cells alter the immune response, particularly the role of monocytes/macrophages. UV light caused apoptosis in autologous peripheral blood lymphocytes (PBLs), while IL-2 deficiency caused apoptosis in murine CTLL-2 cells(Fürnrohr et al., 2005). Monocytes and PBMCs did not generate detectable levels of cytokines in the absence of stimulation. Thus, either heat-aggregated human immunoglobulins that mimic immune complexes or bacterial lipopolysaccharides (LPS), which are strong inducers of cytokine production from monocytes and macrophages, were used to stimulate PBMCs and monocytes. PBMCs and purified monocytes produced significantly more of the anti-inflammatory cytokine interleukin (IL)-10 in the presence of apoptotic cells, but not in the presence of freshly prepared paraformaldehyde-fixed PBLs. However, they produced significantly less of the pro-inflammatory cytokines tumor necrosis factor and IL-12. Measurable levels of cytokines were not released by apoptotic cells themselves. Given that they may be mediated by both human and mouse apoptotic cells, the anti-inflammatory properties of apoptotic cells seem to be conserved across mammalian species.

3.13 Research findings on molecules

When exposed to apoptotic cells, monocytes or PBMCs triggered with heat-aggregated human immunoglobulins rather than LPS likewise produced more IL-10 and less TNF-α, but IL-1 and IL-12 were not detectable in such conditions. However, since unstimulated monocytes cultured with endotoxin-free autologous serum produced almost no detectable amounts of cytokines, regardless of the presence of apoptotic cells, the mere presence of apoptotic cells may not be enough to induce IL-10 expression in monocytes. It is possible that even non-activated monocytes might generate trace levels of IL-10, below ELISA detection threshold, but still have a huge biological impact. Human monocyte-derived macrophages can produce high levels of IL-10 due to the presence of apoptotic cells. In the presence of apoptotic cells, researchers also found a substantial reduction in LPS-induced IL-1 and TNF-α production using human monocyte-derived macrophages. The addition of apoptotic cells resulted in a large increase in IL-10 secretion; however, this was somewhat dependent on the experimental situations. After phagocytosing apoptotic neutrophils, researchers found that in vitro differentiated monocyte-derived macrophages released less granulocyte macrophage colony-stimulating factor (GM-CSF), leukotriene C4, thromboxane B2, IL-1, IL-8, and IL-10 when activated by LPS(Balhara & Gounni, 2012). There was an increase in the synthesis of prostaglandin E2, platelet-activating factor (PAF), and transforming growth factor (TGF)-1. However, apoptotic cells appear to trigger the transcription of pro-inflammatory cytokines in several experiments. The phagocytes that interact with apoptotic cells release pro-inflammatory cytokines like MIP-2, IL-1, and IL-8 in addition to anti-inflammatory cytokines. THP-1 cells treated with phorbol myristate acetate, human monocyte-derived macrophages, Kupffer cells, and alveolar macrophages were found to produce pro-inflammatory cytokines. Thus, it is possible that apoptotic cells can potentially produce a slight pro-inflammatory stimulation that anti-inflammatory signals often neutralize. These contradictory findings could most likely be explained by various experimental configurations. The contamination of apoptotic cells with primary or secondary necrotic cells, which can exhibit pro-inflammatory effects, could be another reason for these findings.

In the presence of apoptotic cells, neutralization of IL-10 mostly restored pro-inflammatory cytokine secretion, while neutralization of TGF-α showed only a slight impact on the pattern of cytokine secretion. These findings suggest that elevated IL-10 secretion and, to a lesser extent, elevated TGF-α activity are the primary causes of the alterations in monocyte cytokine production. These findings do not, however, rule out the possibility that the presence of apoptotic cells increases TGF secretion and/or activation. It has been demonstrated that macrophage's enhanced TGF production plays a role in the suppression and immunomodulatory effects of apoptotic cells. The contribution of elevated IL-10 secretion in macrophages to the immunomodulatory and anti-inflammatory actions of apoptotic cells is somewhat conflicting, suggesting that the experimental settings may influence the induction of IL-10 secretion from macrophages by apoptotic cells. Using human monocyte-derived macrophages activated with lipopolysaccharide (LPS), some researchers failed to find elevated IL-10 concentrations following macrophage exposure to apoptotic cells. Some researchers found that human or murine macrophages exposed to apoptotic cells, with or without stimulation, had higher levels of IL-10. The immunogenicity of apoptotic tumor cells was significantly elevated in a mouse tumor vaccination model in the case of IL-10 deficient mice, indicating that IL-10 appears to be essential for mediating the immunosuppressive effects of apoptotic cells in vivo. Since anti-TGF-β1 antibodies or PAF receptor antagonists restored the cytokine production of LPS-activated macrophages that had been exposed to apoptotic cells, TGF-β1, prostaglandin E2, and PAF appeared to be involved in the inhibition of pro-inflammatory cytokine secretion in monocyte-derived macrophages. There is evidence of other mechanisms that directly suppress the production of pro-inflammatory cytokines in monocytes/macrophages exposed to apoptotic cells, in addition to the paracrine regulation of pro-inflammatory cytokine production. In contrast to macrophages cultured with identical antibodies but without apoptotic cells, the addition of neutralizing antibodies to IL-10 and TGF-β could not fully restore cytokine secretion, either alone or in combination. Two hours after LPS activation, some researchers reported an instantaneous suppression of TNF-α and IL-6 release in macrophages exposed to apoptotic cells. These findings imply that apoptotic cells directly and instantly reduce inflammation in the engulfing macrophage. There is convincing evidence that apoptotic cells actively inhibit pro-inflammatory responses by monocytes and macrophages in addition to passively avoiding them.

3.14 Multiple receptor involvement

Antibodies (LM609) or RGD peptides that engaged the vitronectin receptor v3, decreased the anti-inflammatory effect of apoptotic cells and showed no agonistic activity(Berezin et al., 2014). Even though CD36 ligation replicated the anti-inflammatory properties of apoptotic cells, the alterations in monocyte cytokine secretion patterns brought about by CD^{36} were consistently less potent than those brought about by apoptotic cells. Patients who are genetically mutated to lack the CD^{36} antigen do not exhibit any symptoms of autoimmunity, inflammatory diseases, or poor apoptotic cell clearance. Since many receptor systems mediate the engulfment of apoptotic cells, researchers hypothesized that multiple receptors may be transducing the anti-inflammatory signal into monocytes/macrophages. The absorption of apoptotic cells via this unique PS receptor was blocked by PS and its structural analogs, but not by other anionic phospholipids, although other surface molecules with possible PS receptor function have been previously reported. T and B cells were able to identify and engulf apoptotic cells in a PS-specific way when the PS receptor gene was transfected into them. Macrophages were shown to have anti-inflammatory properties when exposed to a monoclonal antibody produced against the PS receptor. As a result, apoptotic cells can transduce an anti-inflammatory signal through at least two receptors.

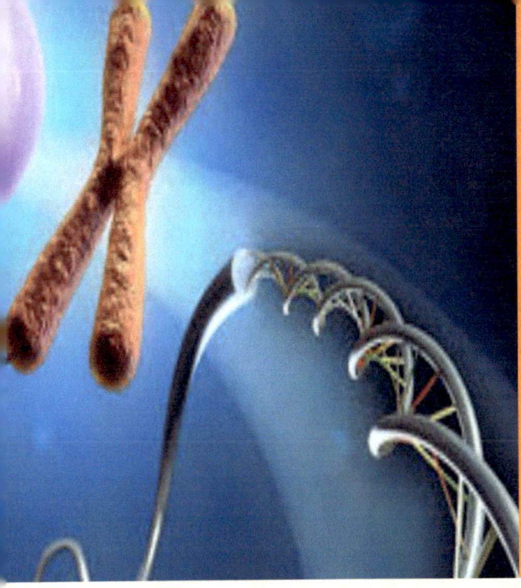

Chapter 4

EPIGENETICS AND DISEASES

Contents

4.1 Introduction

The immune system has a challenging job; to protect the person, it must identify a wide variety of infections while also limiting its ability to identify its own tissues. Lymphocytes can do these tasks by somatically altering their antigen receptor genes. It can create self-reactive cells, which can result in autoimmune disorders if they are not controlled. There are two levels of control over this process: peripheral tolerance and central tolerance.

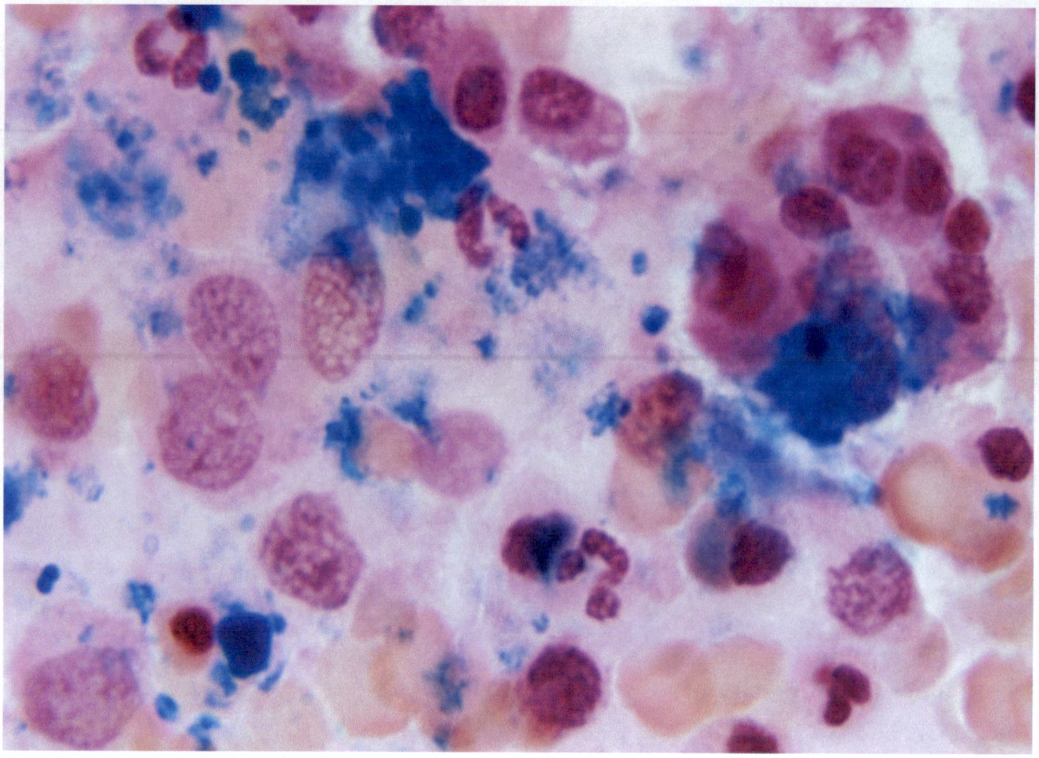

Figure 4.1 Bone marrow

Source: https://upload.wikimedia.org/wikipedia/commons/d/d5/Section_of_bone_marrow_tissue_%28Prussian_blue_stain%29.jpg,Creative Commons License.

From the bone marrow, (Figure 4.1) T cell precursors go to the thymus, where they mature and undergo antigen-recognition-based selection. Apoptosis is triggered and putative self-reactive thymocytes with antigen receptors that bind tightly to self-antigens provided by thymic epithelial and dendritic cells are subjected to negative selection. However, mature T cells with self-reactive T cell receptors (TCRs) may escape to the periphery, and negative selection of self-reactive thymocytes is not entirely successful(Stritesky et al., 2012). T cell activation against self-antigens is restricted by both extrinsic and cell intrinsic mechanisms. Our immune system is good at defending against microbial infections and the development of tumors. However, it needs to be tightly regulated to avoid both accidental aggression by self-reactive immune cells against healthy bodily tissue and tissue damage from immune reactions. The immune system needs to be able to distinguish between dangerous non-self-antigens and harmless self-antigens, maintain immunity against invasive infections, and promote self-tolerance. In order to achieve this, a number of self-tolerance mechanisms have developed. These mechanisms either eliminate lymphocytes that express autoreactive antigen receptors during development and maturation or inactivate and/or delete mature self-reactive cells that have escaped central tolerance mechanisms. It has been hypothesized that a dominant suppression mechanism mediated by a type of suppressor T cell exists in addition to peripheral tolerance mechanisms including clonal deletion, immunological ignorance, and induction of T cell anergy.

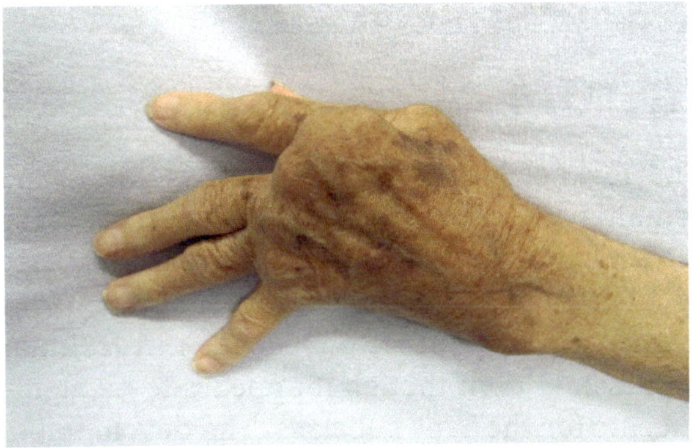

Figure 4.2 Rheumatoid arthritis

Source: https://upload.wikimedia.org/wikipedia/commons/7/70/Rheumatoid_Arthritis.JPG,Creative Commons License.

4.2 Autoimmune conditions

In several autoimmune conditions, including type 1 diabetes, RA or rheumatoid arthritis, (Figure 4.2), and inflammatory bowel disease, Tregs have been demonstrated to have a protective role. Because they can be triggered in an antigen-specific pattern, Tregs have therapeutic applications. They may reduce autoimmune reactions while maintaining protective immunity against pathogen-derived antigens. This characteristic makes them an attractive target for cellular treatment strategies. It appears that Tregs are engaged in a wide range of immunological responses, which means they could potentially be used in various therapeutic applications. Protocols for the in vivo induction of allergen-specific Tregs are presently being developed, as Tregs have also been demonstrated to reduce allergic reactions. Tregs are crucial even during protective immunity against infections, since they have been demonstrated to control pro-inflammatory immune responses to avoid tissue damage and to stop the reaction after the pathogen has been effectively eliminated. Because they prolong the availability of antigens by slowing down or even blocking the pathogen clearance, they even appear to aid in the development of an immunological memory. However, Tregs have also been linked to the appearance of chronicity in some infection models; in these cases, deleting or reducing Tregs may be a helpful treatment strategy. Since tumor-associated antigens are frequently self-antigens and Tregsreduce tumor-rejecting responses, this approach also appears to be the preferred one in terms of tumor immunity. Tregs appear to regulate many immunological responses. As a result, adjusting their quantity, functioning, or activation state could either boost or suppress immune responses as necessary and restore equilibrium to the immune system(Javidan et al., 2024).

Different leukocyte types may be suppressed by interactions among Tregs. When compared to cultures without the suppressors, decreased proliferation of activated T cells in cocultures with Tregs indicates suppression of non-regulatory T cells. Interleukin (IL)-2 is not produced by inhibited T cells. The goal of research has been to determine the mechanism by which Tregs carry out their suppressive role. However, it appears that Tregs employ a variety of methods rather than just one to prevent non-regulatory T cell activation and/or effector functions. Other leukocyte subsets are likely also affected. Tregs can thus choose the mechanism of suppression that best suits the type of immune response, the anatomical site of action, and the initiating antigen, making them ready to respond to a variety of conditions. Four types of suppression have been recognized. Tregs activated phenotype allows them to compete for survival factors and deprive their surroundings of cytokines like IL-2 that are necessary for naïve T cell activation. These cells are unable to fully activate and either fail to proliferate or even die through apoptosis. Tregs and their target cell must be near for this process. cAMP, a second messenger that is known to prevent T cell activation and IL-2 production, is abundant in Tregs. It has been demonstrated that Tregs can use gap junctions to transfer cAMP to their target cell as a suppressive mechanism. Tregs have the ability to alter antigen-presenting cell costimulatory molecule production, which makes them less effective at stimulating non-regulatory T cells. A key component of Treg suppressive action is the inhibitory receptor cytotoxic T lymphocyte antigen 4 (CTLA-4), which is produced on Tregs and can interact with B7 molecules on antigen-presenting cells(Mahnke et al., 2007). Evidence from in vivo studies points to the potential role of inhibitory cytokines like IL-10, TGF-β, or IL-35 in Treg-mediated suppression in specific circumstances.

By directly destroying the responder cells, additional soluble substances generated by Tregs, like granzyme B or perforin, may also increase Treg activity. The α-chain of the IL-2 receptor (CD25), which is typically only upregulated in response to activation through the T cell receptor (TCR), is constitutively expressed on the surface of 10-15% of the $CD4^+$ T cell pool in a healthy mouse. The first surface maker for the Treg population was this constitutive expression of CD25. While CD25 is an indicator of Tregs in the normal state, it can be challenging to differentiate them from newly activated non-regulatory T cells, which can proliferate during an infection or an inflammatory response. Humans, who are constantly exposed to infectious agents, have a large number of CD25-expressing cells in their peripheral blood, which makes this particularly problematic. Tregs have also been found to constitutively express other activation markers, including CTLA-4, glucocorticoid-induced tumor necrosis factor receptor (GITR), and OX-40(Schreiber, 2016).

4.3 Transcription factors

The forkhead box transcription factor Foxp3 remains the most accurate marker for Treg identification to date. A significant disadvantage of using Foxp3 to separate essential Tregs from diverse populations is its intracellular expression, even though it appears to be highly specific for the Treg subclass. The development of Foxp3-reporter mouse strains has helped researchers understand the obstacles in the murine system. One significant obstacle to the therapeutic use of human Tregs in clinical settings is the absence of a Treg-specific surface marker. When researchers were investigating the cause of the aggressive autoimmune disease seen in the naturally occurring mouse mutant scurfy, they discovered the Foxp3 gene. The male scurfy mice die of a multiorgan lymphoproliferative disease after developing hyperactive immune responses. They exhibit a frame-shift mutation in exon 8 of the Foxp3 gene, which results in an early stop and truncation of the forkhead box region, making the Foxp3 protein extremely unstable and undetectable. Because Foxp3 is found on the X chromosome, it only affects male hemizygous mice. When Foxp3-knockout mice were produced by targeted gene disruption, the same phenotype was seen, demonstrating that the disease was indeed caused by a lack of Foxp3. Immunodysregulation polyendocrinopathy enteropathy X-linked or IPEX syndrome, a rare but deadly autoimmune disease in young male patients, has also been linked to Foxp3 gene mutations and the lack of functional FOXP3 protein. The symptoms, which are caused by hyper-reactive T cells and resemble the scurfy phenotype in mice, include enteropathy, eczema, thrombocytopenia, type 1 diabetes, anemia, and thyroiditis. These results imply that Foxp3 gene mutations or deletions result in a lack of functional Tregs, which in turn causes peripheral tolerance to break down and cause autoimmunity to develop.

Due to the lack of suppressive Tregs in scurfy-/Foxp3-knockout mice, Foxp3 was thought to be a master switch and lineage-determination factor for Treg production(Polansky et al., 2009). Research has shown compelling evidence that certain Treg aspects can emerge even in the absence of functioning Foxp3, indicating that additional stimuli besides Foxp3 may activate Treg development. However, fully mature peripheral Tregslost the majority of their Treg traits when Foxp3 expression was stopped. Foxp3 appears to function as a lineage-stabilization factor, preserving the Treg identity that was controlled by other signals. However, Foxp3 contributes to Treg function in addition to Treg maintenance. This was demonstrated by Foxp3 over-expression mediated by retroviruses, which gave non-regulatory CD25 $CD4^{+}$ T cells suppressive qualities. When Foxp3 expression was experimentally stopped, peripheral Tregs that were fully functioning lost their ability to suppress. The murine T cells that were stimulated in the presence of TGF-β to temporarily induce Foxp3 expression only showed suppressive action while Foxp3 expression was sustained. When combined, these findings show that Foxp3 is the primary modulator of the suppressive activity of Tregs. At the molecular level, Foxp3 exhibits characteristics of a transcription factor by controlling the amount of transcription of its target genes and binding to DNA through its forkhead box DNA-binding domain. TCR signaling is necessary for binding to DNA. Despite not having a transactivation domain that has been identified, Foxp3 functions as a transcriptional repressor and, on some genes, as a transcriptional activator. Other significant T cell transcription factors, including nuclear factor of activated T cells or NFAT and nuclear factor-kB (NF-kB), have been demonstrated to physically interact with it, impairing its capacity to transactivate its target genes. The inability of Tregsto generate IL-2 following activation, however, is explained by the ability of Foxp3 to outcompete AP-1 and bind with NFAT to an overlapping site in the Il-2 promoter, suppressing Il-2 transcription. Foxp3 target genes have already been mapped. However, more research is needed to determine how these genes affect Treg physiology and function. Extensive studies have also been conducted on the molecular regulation of Foxp3 expression.

4.4 CpG motifs

NFAT and AP-1, two transcription factors that are often triggered in response to TCR-mediated signaling, are necessary for its action(Masuda et al., 1998). It has been observed that Foxp3 transcription is inhibited when the T helper (Th) 2-lineage specification factor GATA3 binds to the promoter. Foxp3 induction appears to be inhibited by the signal transducer and activator of transcription-1 (STAT1) when Th1-polarizing cytokines are present. It appears that IL-2-mediated STAT5 binding increases Foxp3 expression. The Foxp3 gene first intron contains the promoter as well as two additional transcriptionally active enhancer elements. Even after multiple rounds of cell division, purified ex vivo Foxp3+ Tregs that were grown in vitro or adopted into recipient mice that were either lymphogenic or completely immunocompetent showed consistent Foxp3 expression. Given that Foxp3 has been found to be the Treg lineage stability factor, we can propose that epigenetically imprinting this transcription factor expression could guarantee a stable peripheral Treg pool. It has been demonstrated that other T cell subpopulations, such as Th1 and Th2 cells, where the expression of the distinctive cytokines interferon-γ and IL-4 becomes reciprocally imprinted at both gene loci, can also be fixed by epigenetic mechanisms to a particular differentiation phase. Researchers discovered an evolutionarily conserved area in the Foxp3 gene first intron that was rich in CpG patterns, suggesting an epigenetically active element, using in silico analysis. Because intracellular methylases can methylate the cytosine of the CpG dinucleotide and because accidental deamination can cause point mutations by converting a methylated cytosine into a thymidine, CpG motifs are generally underrepresented in the DNA sequence of mammals. Evolution has only conserved CpG motifs in areas where they play a significant role. This is frequently the case in areas involved in gene expression regulation. CpG motifs are unique in this regard since they can exist in either methylation or demethylated forms. When they are methylated, they create a signal for methyl-DNA-binding proteins, which then attract transcriptional co-repressors to suppress gene transcription at nearby loci and start the condensation of low-DNA-accessible chromatin. Certain histone modifications are typically linked to this closed chromatin state, which prevents active transcription.

4.5 Chromatin modifications

The accessible chromatin states with permissive histone modification and active transcription are indicated by demethylated CpG motifs. In addition to this process, methylation at CpG motifs can also affect some transcription factor or TF capacity to bind DNA with recognition sequences that cross these motifs. Methylation-regulated gene expression patterns are transmissible from a parent cell to its daughter cells because DNA methylation patterns are replicated and preserved during cell division. However, because methylation marks can be added or removed upon appropriate signaling, the system is adaptable and can be modified if necessary. Therefore, CpG methylation patterns reflect a level of gene regulation that is independent of the DNA sequence and modifiable, but that is heritable in a particular state. The activation state of the nearby gene loci can be inferred from the methylation state of CpG-rich areas. In contrast to Foxp3 - T cells, which were fully methylated, Tregs displayed complete demethylation on all CpG motifs when researchers compared the methylation pattern of the conserved CpG-rich element in the Foxp3 locus between murine ex vivo isolated Foxp^{3+} CD25^{+}CD4^{+} Tregs and Foxp^{3-} CD25^{-} CD4^{+} T cells(Huehn & Beyer, 2015). A CpG-rich control region in intron 7 of the Foxp3 gene, which was highly methylated in both cell types, did not exhibit such a differential methylation pattern, suggesting that the selective demethylated state of Tregs in the evolutionarily conserved intron-1 element was not a random event. For this reason, researchers called it the Treg-specific Demethylated Region (TSDR). Other areas of the Foxp3 locus, in addition to TSDR, may also play a role in the epigenetic regulation of Foxp3 expression. For instance, the promoter region also contains many CpG motifs. However, Foxp3 T cells also exhibit a high degree of demethylation, whereas Foxp3 Tregs exhibit complete demethylation on all motifs at that site. This suggests that the promoter region is already in a more open chromatin state even in Foxp3 T cells, and that the availability or activity of the necessary transcription factors may regulate transcription initiation more than the accessibility of the promoter region.

The human FOXP3 promoter region has several CpG motifs, similar to the murine counterpart. These motifs are often only weakly methylated, meaning they only marginally differ from the totally demethylated FOXP^{3+} Tregs. When combined, the observation that FoxP3 locus sequences that have evolved over time are fully and specifically demethylated upon differentiation into persistent Tregs points to a significant role in the epigenetic imprint of this trait. It has also been demonstrated that under a variety of tolerogenic conditions, mature CD25^{-} CD4^{+} non-regulatory T cells can be converted to FoxP+ Tregs in the periphery, even though the thymus is likely where the majority of Tregs are produced. Peripheral Treg induction upon oral feeding of a foreign antigen is thought to be the event, and it is most likely a mechanism that supports immune tolerance to food-borne antigens. To circumvent protective immunity, several pathogens appear to induce or increase suppressive T-cell populations. In autoimmune conditions, when more Tregs are desired to reduce undesired immune reactions, these peripheral conversion processes offer a potential target for novel treatment methods. Less is currently understood regarding the function of these in vivo-induced Treg populations, as well as the necessary signals for FoxP3 activation. Activating murine Foxp3- CD25- CD4^{+} T cells via their TCR in the presence of TGF-β provides a simpler and hence more controllable conversion method in vitro(McHugh et al., 2015). After just a few days, cells from these cultures acquire the ability to suppress and turn on Foxp3 expression. Ex vivo-isolated peripheral naïve T cells from patients may be converted into a significant number of Tregs using the TGF-β-driven in vitro conversion mechanism, which could then be returned as Tregsto reduce unwanted immunity. The majority of iTregs lost both Foxp3 expression and suppressive activity upon re-stimulation in TGF-β-free media, indicating that TGF-β-induced Foxp3 expression is unstable and solely dependent on the inducing cytokine. Indeed, those unstable iTregs were nearly fully methylated when researchers examined the methylation status of TSDR. These results supported that Foxp3 expression can be initiated when TSDR is methylation, and that Foxp3 expression stability requires a demethylated state. This was further demonstrated in subsequent studies when they were able to maintain TGF-β-induced Foxp3 expression with the administration of azacitidine, a nucleoside analog that disrupts DNA methyltransferase 1 activity and causes passive DNA demethylation. Foxp3 expression was induced by azacytidine alone when Foxp3- CD25- CD4+ T cells were treated, and this was accompanied by effective Treg specific demethylated region (TSDR) demethylation. Cells treated with azacitidine did not exhibit alterations in the methylation pattern of TSDR, nor did they increase the expression of Foxp3.

4.6 Gene expression patterns

Determining the signals and conditions that might cause demethylation specifically at TSDR and provide a permanent suppressive phenotype without altering the general pattern of gene expression is therefore of significant interest. Although the thymus appears to be the location of these signals, they can also be produced in the periphery under the correct conditions. Researchers were able to gather evidence supporting the latter scenario by examining in vivo-converted Tregs, which were produced by directing the antigen to DEC205+ dendritic cells (Figure 4.3).

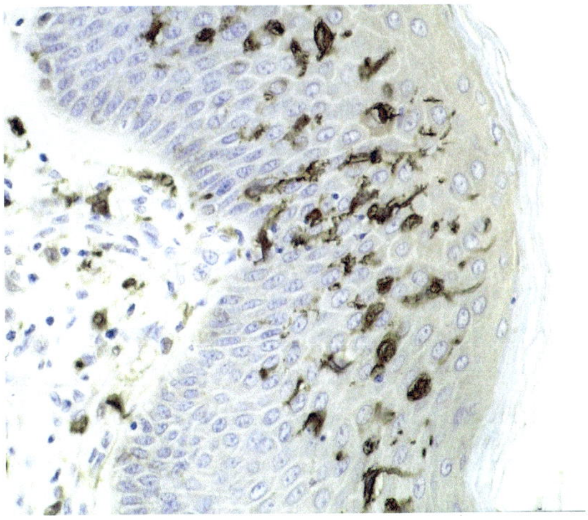

Figure 4.3 DEC205+ dendritic cells

Source: https://upload.wikimedia.org/wikipedia/commons/2/2e/Dendritic_cells.jpg,*Creative Commons License.*

After being restimulated both in vitro and in vivo, the transformed cells showed a high degree of TSDR demethylation and remained stable. It is yet unknown if other in vivo-induced Treg populations such as those produced upon oral feeding also provide a stable phenotype. Even while no long-term tolerance to the eliciting antigen should be developed, it is possible that in some situations only temporary suppressors are required, such as to end a continuing immune response following the removal of a pathogen. Both the intracellular factors that cause or prevent the remodeling of the FoxP3 locus and, in turn, the epigenetic imprinting by demethylation of TSDR, as well as the nature of the determining signal or signals such as the cytokine environment, ligand–receptor binding, and duration of dendritic cell–T cell interaction remain entirely unknown. Some dendritic cell subpopulations may be uniquely suited for the induction and possibly even stabilization of FoxP3 expression in naïve T cells. Medullary thymic epithelial cells (mTECs), (Figure 4.4) which are thought to mediate Treg production or selection, may exert this function in the thymus.

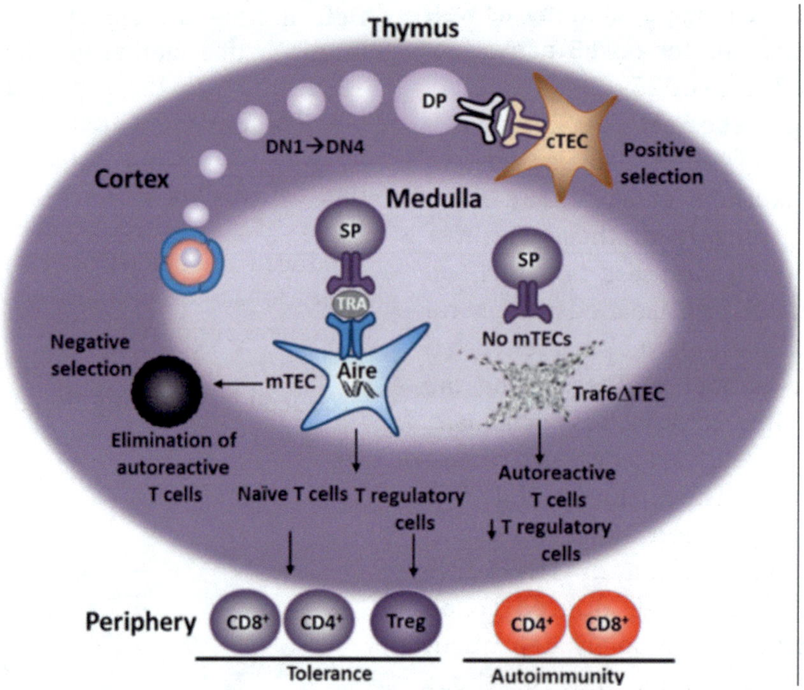

Figure 4.4 Medullary thymic epithelial cells

Source: Alexandropoulos, K., Bonito, A. J., Weinstein, E. G., & Herbin, O. (2015). Medullary Thymic Epithelial Cells and Central Tolerance in Autoimmune Hepatitis Development: Novel Perspective from a New Mouse Model. International Journal of Molecular Sciences, 16(1), 1980-2000. https://doi.org/10.3390/ijms16011980,*Creative Commons License.*

The vitamin A metabolite all-trans-retinoic acid is one soluble molecule that has drawn interest in the Treg sector since it can improve TGF-β-mediated FoxP3 induction in vitro. Although the impact of retinoic acid on the methylation status of TSDR has not yet been examined, human CD25-$CD4^+$ naïve T cells generated from umbilical cord blood treated with retinoic acid experienced histone acetylation at the FOXP3 promoter. This result is consistent with a study that found that adoptive transfer and in vivo re-stimulation improved the FoxP3 stability of Tregs treated with retinoic acid in vitro. These findings support the notion that histone alterations play a role in the epigenetic regulation of FoxP3 expression. FoxP3+ Treg numbers and suppressive activity were raised when histone deacetylase inhibitors were administered in vivo. This resulted in the buildup of acetylated histones, which are typically associated with an open chromatin structure. Acetylated histone 4 accumulated in the FoxP3 promoter region as a result of NFAT and Smad3 binding to the TGF-β-sensitive enhancer region in intron 1(Delacher et al., 2014). Therefore, it appears that in the absence of epigenetic imprinting, which is demonstrated by the demethylated state of the evolutionarily conserved element TSDR, FoxP3 expression and, consequently, the suppressive ability of Tregs, remain transient, even though the mechanisms causing the remodeling of the FoxP3 locus are still unclear.

A family of structurally related transcription factors is known as nuclear factor kB (NF-kB). The five members of the NF-kB family in mammals are c-Rel, RelA (p65), RelB, NF-kB1, and NF-kB2. The 300 amino acid Rel homology domain (RHD), which is structurally conserved in all of them, contains regions that cause dimerization, nuclear translocation, and DNA binding. The transactivation domain, which is non-homologous and found at the C-termini of the proteins, is unique to RelA, RelB, and c-Rel. The seven ankyrin repeats, a 33-amino acid pattern of inhibitor of NF-kB (IkB) that facilitates protein–protein interactions, are present in the other two NF-kB proteins, NF-kB1 and NF-kB2, although lacking a transactivation domain. While the mature forms of RelA, RelB, and c-Rel are expressed, NF-kB1 and NF-kB2 are produced as precursor proteins, p105 and p100, respectively. To keep NF-kB in the cytoplasm, the ankyrin repeats containing NF-kB1 (p105) and NF-kB2 (p100) can act as IkB-like proteins. Proteolytic cleavage and degradation of the ankyrin domain results in the production of the mature versions of NF-kB1 (p50) and NF-kB 2 (p52)(Héron et al., 1995). By homo- or hetero-dimerization, the five NF-kB proteins can create 15 transcription factors. Although p50 and p52 homodimers can bind to DNA, their absence of a transactivation domain causes them to behave as transcription repressors. But when they attach to the IkB-like protein Bcl-3, they can activate transcription.

The two primary NF-kB activated variants are RelA:p50 and RelB:p52. Members of the NF-kB family are essential for many biological functions, such as development, cell proliferation, apoptosis, immunological and inflammatory responses, and more. IkB proteins, which are specific inhibitors that bind RHD through the ankyrin domain and cover the nuclear localization signal function of NF-kB, keep NF-kB dimers inactive in the cytoplasm of resting (dormant) cells.

4.7 Activation pathways

Either p100 processing in the alternative pathway or IkB degradation in the conventional pathway can activate NF-kB dimers. The two main NF-kB dimers that the canonical pathway activates are RelA:p50 and c-Rel:p50. Processing of p100, a protein that can heteromerized and sequester RelB, RelA, and c-Rel, is necessary for the activation of RelB: p50 since it is normally sequestered by p100. The RelB:p52 heterodimer is created and activated when p100 is processed to p52. Even while RelA:p52 and c-Rel:p52 heterodimers are also generated, they are regulated by several IkB inhibitors, primarily IkBa and IkBb, whose breakdown necessitates IkB kinase (IKK) activation, as in the conventional pathway. As a result, these NF-kB dimers are located at the intersection of alternative and canonical NF-kB pathways, a situation known as a hybrid pathway.

Many stimuli can activate the canonical route or pathway. Strong inducers of the classical NF-kB pathway include pro-inflammatory stimuli like pathogen-derived lipopolysaccharide and cytokines like interleukin or IL-1 and tumor necrosis factor a (TNF-α). IKK is activated in response to stimulation, phosphorylating some serines in the IkB proteins, which causes their ubiquitination and degradation. This permits the release and nuclear translocation of NF-kB dimers, which in turn triggers the activation of genes. This pathway primarily activates the NF-kB dimer RelA:p50, which causes the expression of several innate immune and inflammatory genes to coordinate(Basak & Hoffmann, 2008). The activation of the canonical NF-kB route or pathway is IkB degradation. The ankyrin repeats found in IkBs, a class of structurally related proteins, interact with the nuclear-localizing signals of RHDs to stop the nuclear translocation of Rel subunits. The way that different IkBs interact with NF-kB dimers varies. IkBa, for instance, binds to a complex that contains RelA or c-Rel but not to dimers that contain RelB or to p50 or p52 homodimers. Further, p50:p50 and p52:p52 homodimers are the ones that Bcl-3 preferentially binds to. The p50 subunit is preferentially bound by IkBz, the most recently discovered IkB. The transcriptional selectivity of target genes may be partially produced by the complexes that form between IkBs and NF-kB dimers. IkB degradation is dependent on ubiquitin and proteasomes. The phosphorylation of IkB, which starts the ubiquitin-proteasome degradation pathway, depends on IKK. IKKβ (NEMO), a structural subunit, and two kinase subunits, IKKα and IKKβ, make up the IKK complex(Z. J. Chen, 2012). IKKb is crucial of the two kinase subunits for the classical NF-kB pathway to be activated, but the canonical NF-kB activity appears to be unaffected by the absence of IKKα. The NF-kB pathway cannot be canonically activated without IKKγ. Because activation could lead to harmful or even fatal disorders like acute inflammation, septic shock, cell hyperplasia, and cancer, the canonical NF-kB pathway must be regulated and quickly stopped after stimulation. The process involves the production of IkBs, which enter the nucleus, bind to NF-kB dimers, and then return to the cytoplasm to stop the transcription of genes that cause inflammation. Two other processes are also used to guarantee the effectiveness of this feedback inhibition: deacetylation of Rel proteins, which promotes IkB binding, and inactivation of IKK activity, which protects freshly generated IkBs.

Another target for NF-kB activity control is ubiquitination, which is crucial for the activation of NF-kB pathways. The purposes of various ubiquitination may vary. The ability of Lys-48-linked polyubiquitination to make proteins susceptible to proteasomal degradation is its common function. On the other hand, Lys-63-linked polyubiquitin chains or mono-ubiquitination primarily control protein kinase activity and protein transport, including endocytosis and lysosomal targeting. A20 and cylindromatosis (CYLD) are the two deubiquitinating enzymes that have been found to have significant roles in controlling the NF-kB pathway by altering the ubiquitination profile. While CYLD cleaves Lys-63-linked polyubiquitin chains from many proteins, including TNF-receptor-associated factor (TRAF)2, TRAF6, and NF-κB essential modulator (NEMO), to prevent NF-kB activation, A20 participates in two functions(Courtois & Fauvarque, 2018). RIP or TRAF6 activation is prevented by breaking down Lys-63-linked polyubiquitin chains and reassembling Lys-48-linked polyubiquitin chains on RIP for proteasomal degradation. Through physical interaction, additional inhibitory molecules including Twist and protein inhibitor of activated STAT-1 (PIAS1) can also block RelA transactivation activity. It is interesting to note that whereas NF-kB activation can induce Twist expression, PIAS1 cannot. However, IKKα-activated pro-inflammatory stimuli are necessary for PIAS1 phosphorylation, which is necessary for its repressive activity. Non-inflammatory triggers like lymphotoxin β (LTβ) signaling, receptor activator of NF-kB ligand (RANKL), CD40L, and B cell-activating factor belonging to the TNF family (BAFF) typically initiate the non-canonical or alternative pathway. It has been demonstrated that the expression of genes essential to the growth, upkeep, and operation of primary and secondary lymphoid organs is mostly regulated by the alternative NF-kB pathway. IKKβ and IKKγ are not necessary for the alternative NF-kB pathway to be activated; NF-kB-inducing kinase (NIK) and IKKα are the only requirements. IKKβ phosphorylates IkBα more effectively than IKKα and NKIK does not phosphorylate it. In addition to activating IKKα, NIK also attracts IKKα to the p100 complex, at which it phosphorylates the N- and C-terminal serines of p100, causing p100 to be ubiquitinated and undergo further processing. As a result, the protein kinase NIK serves as an adapter molecule as well. It is also crucial to remember that the processing-inhibitory domain (PID domain)-mediated intrinsic inhibition is lessened by NKI-mediated phosphorylation of p100 at serines 866 and 870.

Since RelB is frequently linked to the RHD of p100, activation of this alternate pathway causes the p52-RelB heterodimer to translocate nuclearly(Fagerlund et al., 2008). The alternative NF-kB pathway is regulated with a p100 processing. The first possibility is that p100 itself has a three-dimensional domain that could trap the C-terminal sequences needed for IKKa recruitment. Second, both trans-acting regulatory molecules and cis-acting sequences can adversely limit NIK activity. The protein-level regulation of NIK activity is possible. According to some research studies, TRAF3 can prevent p100 processing by causing the proteasome to degrade NIK. The heat-shock protein 90 (HSP90) maintains NIK stability and the functional inhibition of HSP90 effectively breaks down its connection with NIK, leading to NIK degradation and p100 processing blockage. It has been demonstrated that the multifunctional cytokine Tweak induces p100 processing through an unidentified mechanism that depends on TRAF2, IKKa, and NIK. The close cross-talk between the conventional and alternative NF-kB pathways helps to fine-tune signaling processes. In addition to upregulating classical IkBs and causing negative feedback, activation of the canonical NF-kB pathway also increases the expression of RelB and p100. As a negative feedback mechanism, p100 can likewise prevent the nuclear translocation of dimers containing RelA, just like classical IkBs. It has been demonstrated that p100 in T cells restricts RelA-mediated NF-kB activity after activation. The elevated RelB expression may also function as a negative feedback mechanism. On the other hand, the homeostasis level of p100 and RelB transcription is decreased when IKKb or RelA are not constitutively active.

It has also been demonstrated that RelA activation inhibits RelB function. RelA can bind to RelB in response to TNF-α stimulation, reducing its trans-activation activity. The phosphorylation of Ser-276 of RelA is necessary for this RelA-RelB connection or association, and without it, TNF-α stimulation causes a significant rise in the expression of endogenous NF-kB-responsive genes(Christian et al., 2016). This complex may act as a negative feedback mechanism to reduce RelA activation. In murine embryo fibroblasts, overexpression of RelB reduces TNF-α-induced RelA activity, while deficiency of RelB leads to elevated and sustained RelA activity and responsive gene expression. However, as IkBα stability is similarly decreased in the absence of RelB, the underlying processes of RelB-mediated suppression may involve more than just the creation of the RelA-RelB complex. Presenting TRAs to developing thymocytes to negatively select organ-specific autoreactive thymocytes is one of the key roles of medullary thymic epithelial cells (mTEC). Both autoimmune regulator (AIRE)-dependent and independent mechanisms regulate the thymic expression of tissue-restricted antigens (TRAs). One common abnormality shared by all of the mutant animals is decreased thymic expression of AIRE/TRA. It is uncertain how NF-kB activity contributes to the cell autonomous regulation of AIRE/TRA. Thymocytes at the DP stage are subject to both positive and negative selection, and the key factor influencing the outcome of DP thymocytes is the TCR affinity for the self-peptide-MHC complex(Fink & Bevan, 1995). Because of a process known as positive selection, those with low affinity will multiply. High-affinity DP thymocytes either differentiate into regulatory T cells or are subjected to negative selection. By rearranging additional TCR gene loci to create a new TCR, a process known as receptor editing, thymocytes can occasionally save failed positive selection.

4.8 NF-kB

NF-kB typically binds to inhibitory proteins (IkB) to be sequestered in the cytoplasm. TCR activation can cause IkB to degrade and NF-kB to go to the nucleus, where it performs its transcriptional activity(Zinatizadeh et al., 2021). Nuclear translocation of RelA, RelB, and c-Rel in response to TCR interaction and TNF-α may be eliminated by overexpressing an active super-inhibitory version of IkBa. Normal negative selection but impaired positive selection is observed in transgenic mice producing a mutant version of IkBa. It appears that the sole positive selection impact is $CD8^+$ SP. This selective necessity of NF-kB on CD8+ SP positive selection was also validated by some investigations employing transgenic mice overexpressing a different mutant version of IkBa. These studies also discovered that NF-kB activity is higher in $CD8^+$ SP thymocytes than in $CD4^+$ SP thymocytes. There may be multiple levels of the underlying processes of NF-kB activity in thymocyte positive selection. NF-kB is thought to be pro-apoptotic during negative selection, despite appearing to have an anti-apoptotic function during thymocyte positive selection. Due to negative selection, DP thymocytes are mostly lacking in male H-Y-specific TCR transgenic mice. Since this population is intact in female H-Y TCR transgenic mice, which lack negative signaling to self-antigens, this is not the result of impaired positive selection. However, the male mice DP thymocytes are partially saved if an IkB super-repressor partially inhibits NF-kB. This provides evidence for NF-kB proapoptotic function in negative selection. Some studies suggested that NF-kB might play a different role and that negative selection requires NF-kB suppression. Peptides that cause negative selection upregulate IkBNS, a new IkB-like NF-kB inhibitor, but not peptides that cause positive selection or non-selecting peptides. NF-kB reporter transcription is blocked by IkBNS. TCR-triggered cell death is enhanced by retroviral transduction of IkBNS in fetal thymic organ culture, which is consistent with its role in selection. The function of IkBNS in thymocyte negative selection has to be verified using a physiological model. Depending on the situation and timing, it has been proposed that NF-kB may play a role in thymocyte negative selection that is both pro- and anti-apoptotic. The H-Y TCR or a superantigen-specific TCR was used as a model system in the majority of investigations on NF-kB and thymocyte selection. Therefore, it is yet unknown if and how NF-kB pathways contribute independently to the development of central tolerance against TRAs.

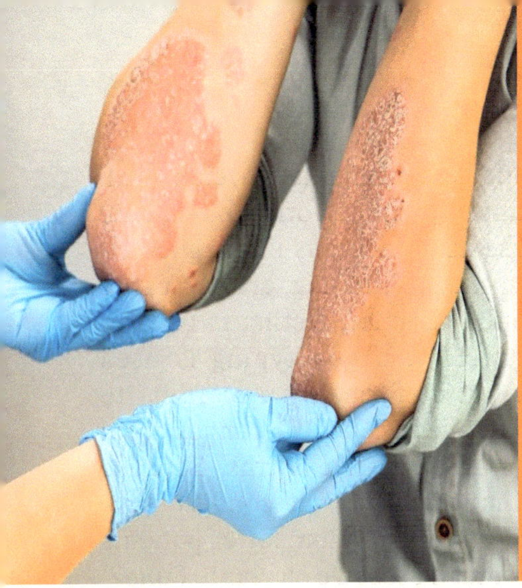

Chapter 5
FUNGAL DISEASES

Contents

5.1 Introduction

In patients suffering from primary or acquired immunodeficiency, invasive fungal infections, or IFIs, are important causes of morbidity and mortality. Depending on the type of immunological problems, a wide range of invasive mold and yeast infections are implicated in different ways. Early diagnosis of IFIs is still difficult. Clinical evidence, microbiological analysis, and host variables are used to establish the diagnosis. Diagnostic evaluation has been enhanced by developments in high-resolution radiological imaging and molecular diagnostic techniques. Over the last few decades, the group of antifungal drugs has grown significantly. Several criteria, including risk stratification, local fungal epidemiology patterns, comorbidities, drug interactions, past antifungal use history, and the pharmacologic profile of the antifungal drugs, must be carefully taken into account before beginning antifungal treatment. Primary immunodeficiency disease refers to a collection of diverse diseases brought on by hereditary immune system abnormalities. Many distinct and pleiotropic immune defects have been identified, depending on which immune system component is impacted. These include disorders brought on by phagocytic and complement defects, humoral immune deficiencies, and immunodeficiencies of lymphocytes and natural killer (NK) cells. More than 80% of cases of primary immunodeficiencies are identified(Notarangelo, 2010). These individuals may exhibit recurrent, prolonged, or potentially fatal infections brought on by common pathogens or by opportunistic agents, such as fungi. IFIs are more prevalent and severe in patients with innate defects of the macrophage/monocyte axis, with or without defects in T-cell function, since a successful host immune response against fungal organisms depends on the coordinated contribution of both innate and adaptive immunity. Chronic granulomatous disease (CGD) is a genetic condition characterized by bacterial and fungal infections and excessive inflammatory reactions leading to granuloma development. Nicotinamide adenine dinucleotide phosphate (NADPH) oxidase abnormalities in phagocytes, either absent or malfunctioning, are the cause of CGD. Neutrophil function testing is used to make the diagnosis, and genotyping is used to locate the exact abnormality. According to estimates, the frequency of CGD ranges from 1/200,000 to 1/250,000 live births. Because the majority of mutations in the condition are X-linked, it primarily affects men; fewer patients have an autosomal recessive variant. Fungal infections are most common in CGD, the main immunodeficiency.

5.2 Fungi

Aspergillus species and Candida species and other fungi are responsible for the majority of IFIs in individuals with CGD. Since the introduction of itraconazole prophylaxis and the use of voriconazole and posaconazole for the treatment of filamentous fungal infections (Aspergillus), the frequency of and mortality from IFIs has significantly decreased.

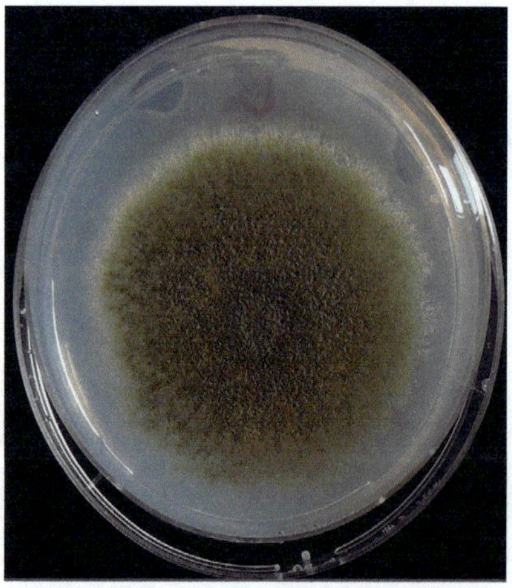

Figure 5.1 *Aspergillus nidulans*

Source: https://upload.wikimedia.org/wikipedia/commons/0/09/Aspergillus_nidulans_wildtype.jpg,*Creative Commons License.*

Although a considerable decrease in the incidence of major infections and mortality is still debatable, the long-term preventive administration of interferon (IFN)-γ in patients with CGD seems to be safe. IFIs are still the most common cause of infectious death in CGD, despite the extensive use of triazole prophylaxis. Aspergillus species are a major cause of death, accounting for one-third of all mortalities. The two most often isolated species are *Aspergillus fumigatus* and *Aspergillus nidulans* (Figure 5.1).

Infections with *A. nidulans* are rarely documented in other immunocompromised patients, suggesting a special relationship between this fungus and the host of CGD and potentially more serious consequences than those of *A. fumigatus*. Although chronic lymphatic and cutaneous involvement has also been reported, the most impacted organs are the lungs, liver, and bones. Routine chest imaging is recommended in the majority of IPA cases. Serum indicators like 1,3-β-D-glucan and galactomannan have limited use in CGD. Segmental and multilobar consolidation, perihilar infiltrates, peripheral nodular masses, numerous tiny nodules, and pleural effusions are among the radiographic manifestations of pulmonary disease. Itraconazole has been used routinely for prophylaxis for nearly 20 years, while posaconazole might be a better option(Copley et al., 2020).

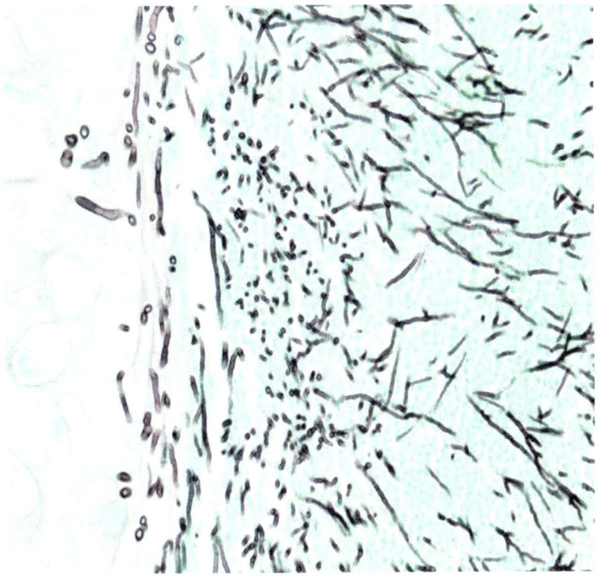

Figure 5.2 Aspergillosis

Source: https://upload.wikimedia.org/wikipedia/commons/6/63/Pulmonary_aspergillosis_%281%29_invasive_type.jpg,*Creative Commons License.*

5.3 Antifungal drugs

Prolonged regimens of antifungal drugs are usually necessary for the management of IA (Invasive aspergillosis) (Figure 5.2). In certain situations, surgery might be necessary for full recovery, particularly when osteomyelitis or infections brought on by *A. nidulans* are present. Other treatments could be taken into consideration as supplemental therapy in cases of IA that are life-threatening.

Granulocyte transfusion from healthy donors may help improve the patient's prognosis by partially restoring their compromised phagocytic activity(Gea-Banacloche, 2017). Although its efficacy is debatable, IFN-γ has also been utilized in a few cases as an adjuvant therapy of IA in CGD patients. The sole treatment for CGD is HSCT (Hematopoietic stem cell transplantation), which may be suitable for some individuals with refractory IA. In the CGD community, Candida is regarded as a rare pathogen. A variety of antifungal medications, such as amphotericin B, azoles, and echinocandins, have been used to treat Candida infections in people with CGD.

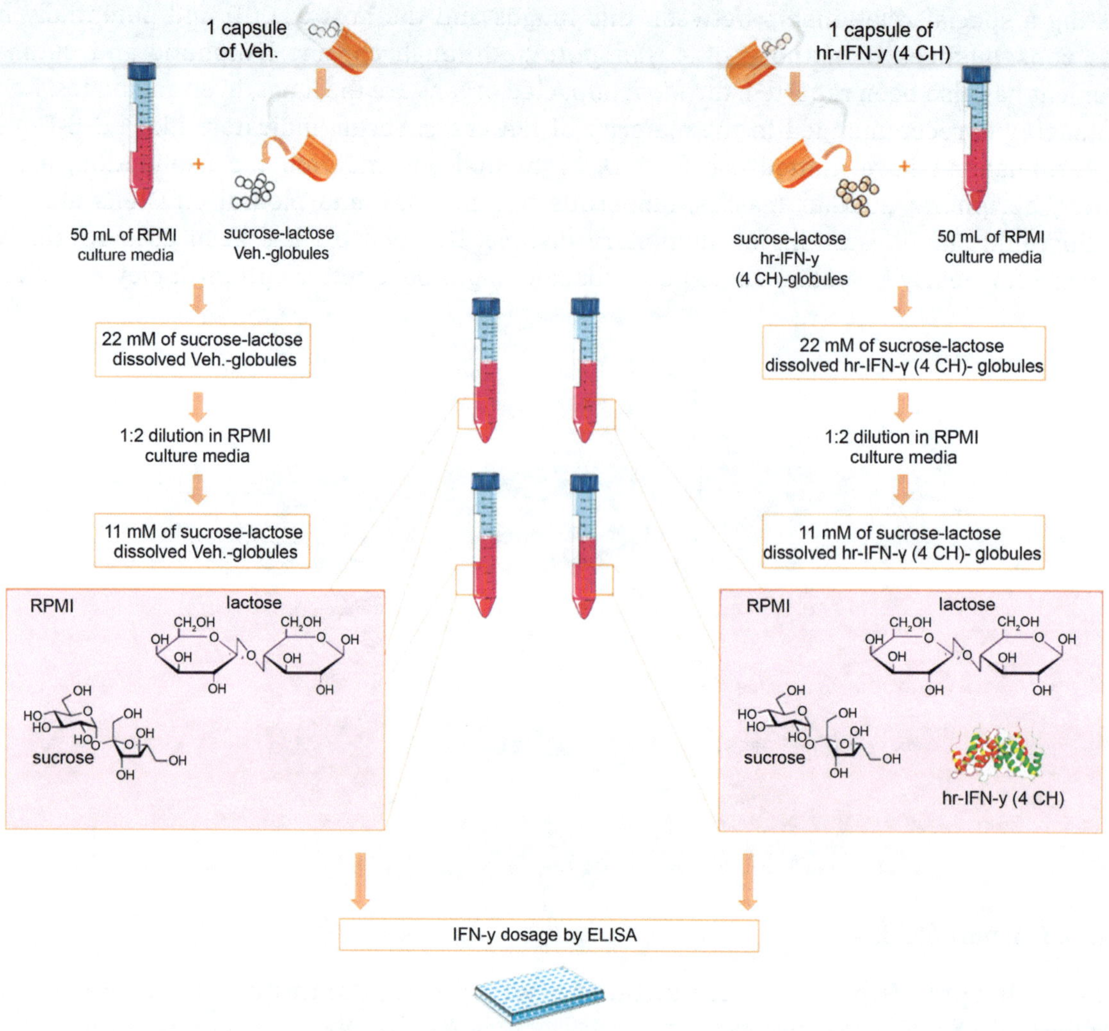

Figure 5.3 IFN-γ immunotherapy

Source: Jacques, C., Chatelais, M., Fekir, K., Brulefert, A., & Floris, I. (2022). The Unitary Micro-Immunotherapy Medicine Interferon-γ (4 CH) Displays Similar Immunostimulatory and Immunomodulatory Effects than Those of Biologically Active Human Interferon-γ on Various Cell Types. International Journal of Molecular Sciences, 23(4), 2314. https://doi.org/10.3390/ijms23042314,*Creative Commons License.*

IFN-γ immunotherapy (Figure 5.3) has also been suggested as a preventative or adjuvant treatment for IC in patients with CGD(Nami et al., 2019). Other fungal species, such as Acremonium, Penicillium, Fusarium, Chrysosporium, and Alternaria, have also occasionally been documented to induce IFIs in patients with CGD. Over 95% of patients with myeloperoxidase MPO deficiency have no symptoms at all. The most commonly reported infections among the small number of MPO-deficient patients with clinical symptoms are caused by various strains of Candida. Sepsis and infections of the mucosa, meninges, and bones have been reported. Other comorbidities, particularly diabetes mellitus, seem to enhance the risk of developing invasive Candida infections. Prophylactic antifungal treatment is not usually advised. Leukocyte migration to inflammatory areas is a dynamic process that involves several adhesion cascade phases. Leukocytes and endothelial cells that are activated and at rest both express different adhesion molecules. Leukocyte adhesion deficiency (LAD) syndromes are caused by defects in several of these adhesion molecules and are usually identified early in the neonatal period. LAD I involves a deficiency or defect in the β-2-integrin family. LAD II involves the absence of fucosylated carbohydrate ligands for selectins. LAD III involves a defect in the activation of all β-integrins; and LAD IV involves a deficiency in Rac2 or Ras-related C3 botulinum toxin substrate 2, which regulates NADPH oxidase and the actin cytoskeleton(Wintergerst et al., 2017).

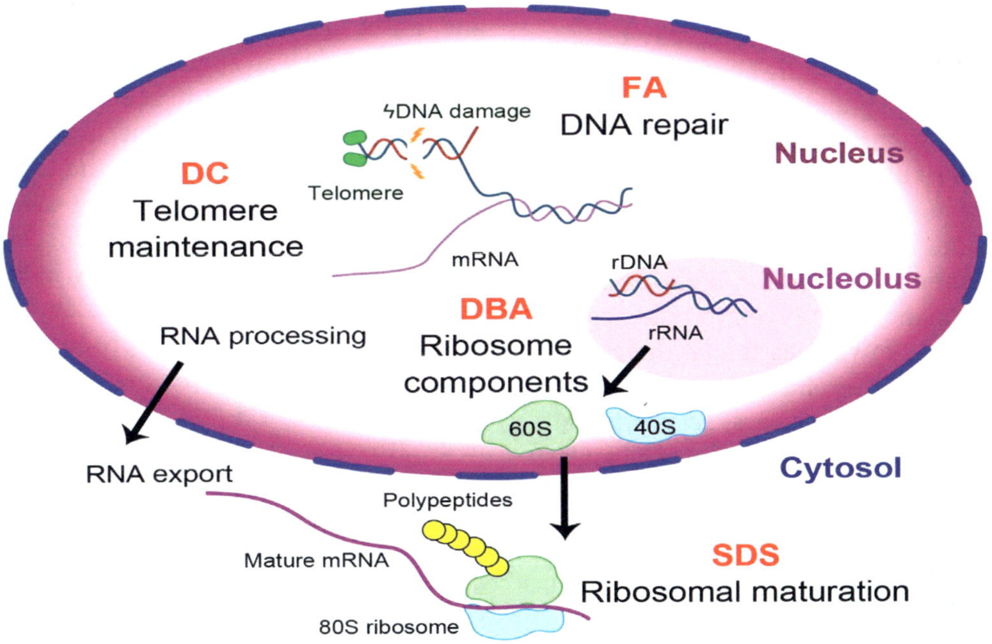

Figure 5.4 Shwachman-Diamond syndrome

Source: Kawashima, N., Bezzerri, V., & Corey, S. J. (2023). The Molecular and Genetic Mechanisms of Inherited Bone Marrow Failure Syndromes: The Role of Inflammatory Cytokines in Their Pathogenesis. Biomolecules, 13(8), 1249. https://doi.org/10.3390/biom13081249,*Creative Commons License.*

5.4 Syndromes

Congenital neutropenia is caused by a primary bone marrow failure syndrome that begins at or around birth. It mostly relates to three conditions: Shwachman-Diamond syndrome (Figure 5.4), cyclic neutropenia, and severe congenital neutropenia. It is interesting to note that IFIs are uncommon in patients with prolonged neutropenia whose other immune functions remain unaltered. However, there have been a few documented cases of IFIs brought on by Aspergillus species, Candida species, and mucormycosis. Recombinant human granulocyte colony-stimulating factor (G-CSF) treatment raises neutrophil counts and lowers the risk of serious infections; HSCT is recommended if G-CSF is not responsive. In immunocompetent people, the majority of fungi that we are frequently exposed to through the air or that are a normal component of our microbiota typically do not cause disease. However, if the host defenses are compromised, certain fungi can turn pathogenic, exhibiting symptoms that range from minor infections to serious systemic diseases that have a high rate of morbidity and mortality. Gaining insight into the immune system's reaction to fungal infections is crucial for creating more effective treatment and prevention strategies. The host reaction to various fungal infections, however, is just as varied and unique as the many fungal diseases. Over the years, scientific and clinical research has uncovered key molecular and cellular factors in host-fungal interactions and host defense, as well as new insights into the pathophysiology of fungi. The majority of fungal infections are brought on by organisms that are either a typical part of our microbiota or to which we are frequently exposed through the air. Usually, they don't make immunocompetent people sick. However, if the host's defenses are compromised, certain fungi can turn harmful, exhibiting symptoms that range from minor superficial infections to serious systemic diseases that have a high rate of morbidity and mortality. Predisposing factors include acquired immunodeficiencies, such as those brought on by HIV infection, antibiotic treatment, or the use of medical devices, as well as immunosuppression caused by corticosteroids or chemotherapy in transplant recipients and tumor patients. Recently, there has been increased awareness of hereditary immunodeficiencies as a rare but significant risk factor for fungal infections. Despite affecting over 25% of the population, the clinical significance of fungal infections is frequently underestimated. Recurrent, chronic, and invasive types of disease are more severe and frequently challenging to treat, even though the majority of cases may be managed with available drugs.

5.5 Pathogens

Many diseases, including superficial, allergic, and tissue-invasive disorders are brought on by fungus-related pathogens. They can be categorized based on tissue tropism and the causative fungal agents. The host reaction to these infections varies widely and is contingent upon the fungus species causing the infection. All of the host tissues are susceptible to superficial fungal infections, which include mucosal, cutaneous, and ocular infections. Candida species commonly produce symptoms in otherwise healthy people by affecting the skin, nails, and oral and vaginal mucosa. Even in healthy people, vulvovaginal infections are extremely common; around 70% of women will have at least one episode in their lifetime, and 5-10% will develop chronic or recurrent vulvovaginal candidiasis. Candida infections of the mouth and esophagus are linked to $CD4^+$ T cell abnormalities, like those seen in patients with progressive AIDS(de Repentigny et al., 2004). More recently, chronic mucocutaneous candidiasis (CMC) with cutaneous and mucosal symptoms has been associated with specific abnormalities in the interleukin-17 pathway. Dermatophytes are the common cause of superficial fungal infections while being less researched than Candida species. They cause common ailments including athlete's foot, and nail infections, which are treatable with antimycotics. However, certain immunological deficiencies enable the development of more severe and occasionally fatal types of dermatomycoses, such as invasive Exophiala infection and dermatophytosis in people with CARD9 deficiency. Commensal yeasts called *Malassezia* spp. are widely distributed on human skin and have been linked to many skin conditions, including folliculitis, and atopic dermatitis. Fungal keratitis can arise as a result of eye trauma, such as that brought on by thorns and sticks. The most common causes of this disease are Aspergillus, Candida, and Fusarium species. It may cause blindness or vision loss if left untreated. The rural communities are especially impacted. People who wear contact lenses are also at risk. Despite being far less common than superficial fungal infections, deep-seated fungal infections are risky due to their high death rates. Both diagnosing and treating them continue to be difficult. The invasive fungal infections occur in hospital environments and arise when fungus breach the natural defenses of susceptible hosts. Among nosocomial infections, systemic candidiasis is ranked as the fourth most prevalent bloodstream infection. When Candida species enter the body through the skin or the gastrointestinal tract, they circulate into the spleen, liver, and/or kidney, resulting in organ failure and sepsis-like syndromes in critically ill patients. Rare organ-specific infections that target the central nervous system (CNS) can be brought on by specific immunological deficiencies, such as those seen in people with genetic abnormalities in the CARD9 gene. The frequent cause of fungal infections in solid organ donation, *Cryptococcus neoformans*, is responsible for half of all fungal infections in HIV patients. A secondary infection of the central nervous system may arise from the systemic spread of *C. neoformans* from the lung and its passage through the blood-brain barrier. *Pneumocystis jirovecii* is another prevalent respiratory opportunistic infection that causes pneumonia in those with weakened immune systems, particularly those living with HIV/AIDS.

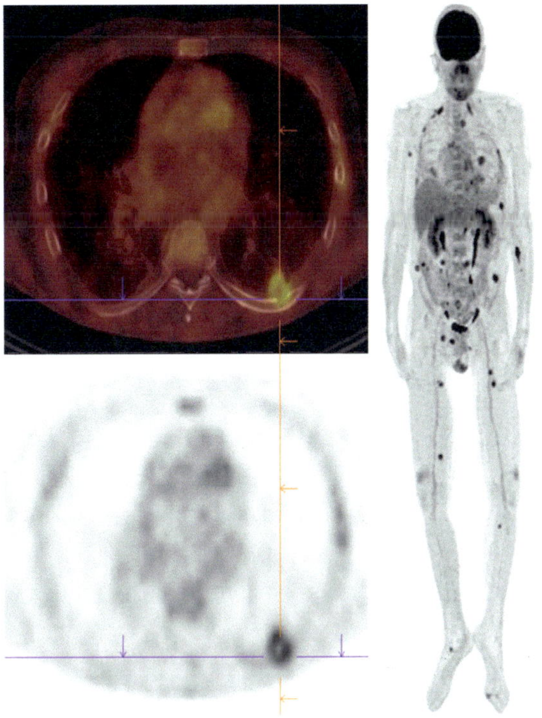

Figure 5.5 Pulmonary aspergillosis

Source: Ledoux, M. -P., & Herbrecht, R. (2023). Invasive Pulmonary Aspergillosis. Journal of Fungi, 9(2), 131. https://doi.org/10.3390/jof9020131,*Creative Commons License.*

Cancer patients, transplant recipients, and those using long-term immunosuppressive medication, such as methotrexate or corticosteroids, are risk categories. Pneumonia patient aerosols or early exposure to family members or neighbors who have the pathogen in their lungs are the two ways that it is spread. Mucormycosis, also known as zygomycosis, is an uncommon but serious fungal disease that arises in leukemia, transplantation, diabetic ketoacidosis, neutropenia, and severe immunosuppression. It is caused by zygomycetes. In this case, angioinvasion causes blood vessel infarction, systemic spread or dissemination, and surrounding tissue necrosis. Up to 80% of transplant recipients may die as a result of their condition. Systemic mycoses are usually caused by thermally dimorphic fungi that are native to specific regions of America(Lockhart et al., 2021).

Persistent exposure to Aspergillus spp. molds can result in invasive pulmonary aspergillosis (Figure 5.5), which has a high fatality rate. Patients with compromised immune systems with low neutrophil counts, recipients of solid organ transplants, patients receiving immunosuppressive treatments, patients with chronic obstructive pulmonary disease (COPD), and patients with cystic fibrosis, are considered to be at risk. Non-immunocompromised patients with past or present lung disease exhibit several types of chronic pulmonary aspergillosis, a progressive lung disease that causes lung damage. Certain fungus may cause allergies.

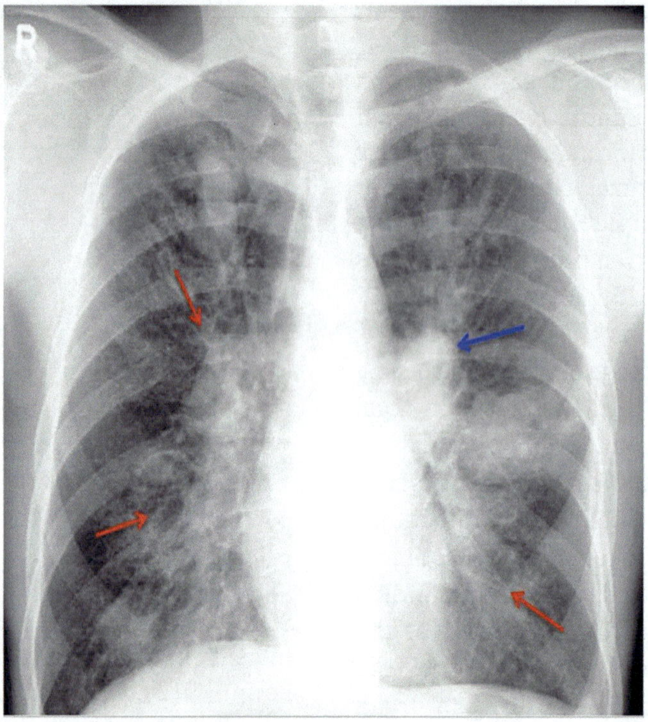

Figure 5.6 Allergic bronchopulmonary aspergillosis

Source: https://upload.wikimedia.org/wikipedia/commons/d/da/Article_river_5800d6205cfa11e99c51c512b70b63f3-Fig-1.png,*Creative Commons License.*

Allergic bronchopulmonary aspergillosis (ABPA) (Figure 5.6) is the most prevalent type of allergy mycosis. Patients with cystic fibrosis and asthma are particularly susceptible to this Th2-mediated allergic disease. The majority of human fungal infections are brought on by commensal or environmental organisms that have coevolved with their host for millions of years without endangering the host in typical conditions. Defects in host defense are the main cause of disease susceptibility. Host mechanisms that preserve homeostasis with various fungus species in various tissue compartments have been identified through research on immunological abnormalities in patients with fungal infections. The epithelium which stops fungal invasion and overgrowth, often maintains fungal control in superficial tissues. The adaptive immune system plays an important role in supporting this function by providing ongoing antigen-specific surveillance and forming memory cells in response to fungal exposure. The acute response of myeloid effector cells of the innate immune system is crucial for defense against invasive and disseminated fungal disease, in which fungi enter the bloodstream and internal organs where they typically do not survive. Mice were used as models for a variety of fungal diseases, and recently, zebra fish models for mucosal and disseminated infections were created. Animal models only partially reflect the situation in humans, although studies on mice significantly improved the investigations.

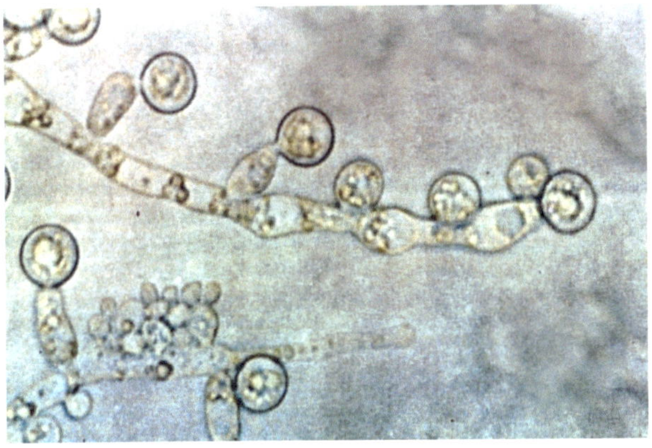

Figure 5.7 *Candida albicans*

Source: https://upload.wikimedia.org/wikipedia/commons/e/e6/Candida_albicans_2.jpg,*Creative Commons License.*

A large number of fungal pathogens, such as *Candida albicans* (Figure 5.7), which are a component of the human microbiome, are typically not commensals in SPF mice. As a result, experimental infections in mice with these species typically represent primary infections that cause acute immune responses; as a result, they differ significantly from human reactions to fungal species. When it comes to surface infections, this difference is significant.

5.6 Virulence

Many pathogenic fungi can change between environmental and pathogenic forms, each of which has a unique virulence potential. Significant alterations in the fungal transcriptional program typically accompany morphotype switching, which modifies the fungal behavior when it comes into contact with the host. The hyphal form is linked to adherence and invasion of host tissue surfaces, although the majority of Candida species are believed to exist as unicellular yeasts conducting asexual reproduction in their commensal condition. In the case of *A. fumigatus*, hyphae are linked to host tissue invasion, and the growth of conidia in the alveolar gaps is accompanied by higher immunogenicity that permits/promotes greater immune system regulation. At least six major human fungal infections are classified as thermally dimorphic fungi, which develop as mold in the soil at room temperature and change into virulent yeast when infectious spores are inhaled(Enoch et al., 2017). The main characteristic of fungal pathogenicity is generally thought to be morphological plasticity rather than a fixed morphotype. During homeostasis and disease induction, epithelial cells are typically the first host cells to come into contact with opportunistic fungal infections. Fungi come into contact with several forms of epithelia, such as simple squamous epithelia (gastrointestinal system and lung) or stratified squamous epithelia (skin and vagina), depending on their tissue tropism. In addition to behaving as simple physical barriers, these epithelia also detect fungi and trigger host defensive responses based on the pathogenicity of the fungus. The research on the relationship between fungi and epithelial cells was conducted on *Candida albicans*. Fungal adherence to the epithelium, invasion, and eventual destruction of epithelial cells are all steps in the passage from *C. albicans* commensalism to infection, which may cause the epithelium to secrete inflammatory mediators. Cell surface adhesins and physical characteristics like cell surface hydrophobicity mediate *C. albicans* attachment to epithelial cells. When *Candida albicans* interact with epithelial cells, several adhesin genes exhibit elevated expression. This function of the Als3 glycosylphosphatidylinositol (GPI)-anchored cell wall protein, which interacts with host cadherins to induce hyphal adhesion, has been established. It is interesting to note that host cell transglutaminases identify Hwp1, another GPI-anchored protein at the *C. albicans* hyphal cell surface that facilitates attachment to epithelial cells and forms a covalent link with host surface proteins. During the yeast-to-hyphae transition, the ALS3 and HWP1 genes, as well as other genes encoding cell surface adhesins involved in the interaction with epithelial cells, are expressed(Fan et al., 2013). This suggests that adhesion is facilitated by this morphotypic switch of *Candida albicans*, while hyphenation is facilitated by adhesion to epithelial cells.

5.7 Cell surface interaction

One crucial stage in the infection process is invasion of the oral epithelium. In the case of *Candida albicans*, it involves aggressive epithelial cell penetration and increased endocytosis. When cell surface proteins or adhesions interact with host cell receptors, such as Als3-cadherin and Ssa1-cadherin interactions, clathrin and other endocytosis components are recruited at the site of interaction between the hyphal tip and the host cell, resulting in induced endocytosis. Other fungi also exhibit actin-dependent endocytosis, as seen in the internalization of *A. fumigatus* conidia by lung epithelial cells. Less is known about how *C. albicans* actively penetrates epithelial cells, however, it may be a combination of mechanical pressure and secreted aspartyl proteases (SAPs). E-cadherin, a component of epithelial tight junctions, has been shown to be degraded by Sap5. *A. fumigatus* hyphae cultured on a human lung sample also showed active penetration, invading across epithelial cells to cause cell injury, cilia loss, and cell detachment. Fungal infections use several ways to connect with endothelial cells to invade during dissemination. The fungus enters the bloodstream through transendothelial migration and then quickly leaves the circulation to enter target organs like the kidney in systemic infection with Candida albicans. In vitro, endothelial cells absorbed *Candida albicans*. Yeast-to-hyphae transition is not necessary for *C. albicans* endothelial transmigration, as evidenced by the findings that in vivo endothelial transmigration into the tissues occurs in minutes, morphological switching occurs over several hours, and yeast-locked *C. albicans* can also enter the tissue. Members of the Als family and Ssa1 bind to N-cadherin on endothelial cells, while αMβ2 integrin-like adhesins probably attach to ICAM-1. These factors are also involved in *C. albicans* adherence and invasion of the endothelium. Zygomycetes have been demonstrated to attach to and be absorbed by endothelial cells in vitro. It is believed that this procedure is essential for zygomycetes to enter blood vessels during pulmonary infections.

Epithelial and endothelial damage results from fungal hyphae invading tissue. Damage to host cells seems to be caused by a variety of methods. The fungal viability alone is insufficient for damage induction. It is also not directly related to invasion. Many genes involved in yeast-to-hyphae transition are necessary for damage induction. It has been observed that SAPs affect E-cadherins in *C. albicans*, which in turn alters the integrity of the epithelium. Recently, it was shown that the

ECE1 gene contributes to epithelial damage by the proteolytic processing of the hyphal-specific Ece1 protein, which results in the extracellular release of peptides, including the candidalysin peptide, which is toxic to host cell membranes. At low doses, candidalysin peptide initiates a risk response pathway that is dependent on c-Fos and MKP; yet, at greater concentrations, it creates pores in epithelial cells that permit calcium influx and cause direct tissue damage(Altmeier & LeibundGut-Landmann, 2017). The production of Ece1 and candidalysin may help to explain why damage to epithelial cells is largely caused by prolonged hyphal development. Therefore, it appears that fungal pathogenicity is directly related to its ability to inflict damage. Epithelium actively reacts and can distinguish between pathogenic and nonpathogenic forms in addition to acting as a crucial physical barrier to stop fungal invasion. Toll-like receptors (TLRs) and dectin-1 are examples of pattern recognition receptors (PRRs) that are expressed by epithelial cells. The fungal identification by epithelial cells also involves PRR-independent signaling pathways. While downstream signaling components were identified, the precise nature of the receptors connecting fungal detection by epithelial cells to cytokine production is yet understood. Although *C. albicans* yeast cells can actually cause basal NFκB and c-Jun activation, their hyphae initiate a profound MAPK response that phosphorylates MPK1 and c-Fos and activates PI3K/Akt/mTOR, leading to the release of cytokines such as G-CSF, GM-CSF, IL-6, and IL-1α.

5.8 Signaling pathways

Individual signaling pathways and the type of epithelial cells determine the quantitative and qualitative variations among various cytokines. It has recently been determined that the candidalysin peptide, which is generated from the hyphal-specific virulence factor Ece1, is a crucial component of *Candida albicans* that initiates these reactions. It was demonstrated that low concentrations of candidalysin induced the secretion of G-CSF and GM-CSF, whereas larger quantities were necessary for the development of pores in the epithelial cells, which subsequently resulted in the release of IL-1α. Epithelial cells produce IL-1α, and it is believed that causing cellular injury is enough to trigger its release. The epithelial response to *A. fumigatus* has also been linked to MAPK signaling, much like the case with *C. albicans*(Yin et al., 2022). Leukocytes like neutrophils, monocytes, and T lymphocytes are drawn to the infection site by cytokines and chemokines produced by epithelial cells. Neutrophils are pleiotropically affected by G-CSF. To fulfill the increased demand for neutrophils during infection and inflammation, it mobilizes neutrophils from the bone marrow and is a crucial regulator of granulopoiesis. Further, G-CSF stimulates Mcl-1 RNA to support neutrophil survival. G-CSF improves neutrophil function, for example, by generating ROS, and it may increase human neutrophil ability to kill *A. fumigatus* and *Candida albicans*. GM-CSF improves neutrophil activity and survival. Together with the related member IL-1β, which is also produced by leukocytes and epithelial cells, at least in humans, IL-1α can work in an autocrine way or paracrine way on epithelial cells to increase the production of cytokines and chemokines, which in turn can stimulate the inflammatory response.Further, IL-1α promotes neutrophil recruitment by producing CXCL1 during acute lung aspergillosis and increases neutrophil activity against the fungus. IL-1R signaling was linked to fungal control and neutrophil recruitment in the setting of oropharyngeal candidiasis.

One significant source of host defense peptides (HDPs) is epithelial cells. Active peptides, which are produced by proteolytic processing from precursors and typically range in size from 10 to 50 amino acids, are primarily positively charged but may also contain a substantial amount of hydrophobic residues. By inactivating the cytoplasmic targets within microbial cells and causing membrane permeabilization, they either eradicate or stop the growth of infections. Many HDPs have antibacterial properties, but they can also modulate the immune system and encourage immune cell chemotaxis. α- and β-defensins, Cathelicidins, and histatins are the main family of HDPs. Certain HDPs are constitutive, whilst others are induced by inflammatory and microbial stimuli in epithelial cells(van der Does et al., 2019). HDP is not just produced by epithelial cells; neutrophils are a significant source of substances like α-defensins and cathelicidins. Nearly all β-defensins are expressed by epithelial cells, and some are triggered by pathogenic fungi. They differ from α-defensins by having cysteine disulfide bonds. Although the exact mechanism of β-defensin-mediated antifungal activity is unknown, it is thought to be energy-dependent. Direct antifungal activity is exhibited by human β-defensin 2 (hBD2) and hBD3 against *A. fumigatus* and *Candida* spp. Human salivary glands are the only organs that express histatins. During and after secretion, the protein histatin 3 is subjected to several proteolytic cleavages, resulting in cascades of peptide products, including histatin 5 (Hst5). Through binding to *C. albicans* Ssa1 and Ssa2, intracellular translocation, impairment of the fungal Trk1 transporter function, and ultimately ATP and potassium efflux, Hst5 fungicidal activity is dependent on its ability to upset cellular ionic homeostasis. Cell cycle halt and cellular shrinkage are brought on by the depletion of cytosolic ions. Hst5 induces oxidative stress, impacts mitochondrial activities, and may prevent *Candida albicans* from adhering to epithelial cells.

5.9 Cell wall

Cell wall β-1,3-exoglucanase Xog1 was found to bind LL-37 in *Candida albicans*(Ma et al., 2024). This leads to intracellular translocation, substantial disruption of the *Candida albicans* cell membrane, nucleotide and protein efflux, and processing of LL-37 by cell wall proteases. Cramp was thought to be the cause of mice resistance to *C. albicans* colonization. Calprotectin is one example of a metal-chelating agent that can stop fungal development. In response to fungal infection, the calprotectin subunits S100A8 and S100A9 are substantially increased. During barrier tissue infections with *Candida albicans* and *A. fumigatus*, animals lacking S100A9 exhibit poor fungal clearance. The presence of several antimicrobial effectors, many of which appear to have redundant effects, ensures that the host is well protected against a wide range of microorganisms. Therefore, the host's ability to effectively control an infection may not be affected by the absence of a specific antimicrobial effector. Antimicrobial defense peptides that mediate direct antifungal control, alarmins like IL-1α that signal the presence of invasive pathogens, chemotactic factors that can attract immune cells, and cytokines that signal to and activate immune cells are just a few of the ways that epithelial cells respond to infection. Although the fungus directly causes a large number of those reactions, microbially produced cytokines may also intensify them. The epithelium combines host and fungal signals to support effective host defense in barrier tissues. Depending on the route and extent of invasion, fungal pathogens may come into touch (contact) with immune cells in the host tissue as well as in the bloodstream if they manage to get past the first epithelial barrier and begin to infiltrate the tissue. Through germline-encoded PRRs, the innate immune system has developed the ability to detect conserved microbial structures known as pathogen-associated molecular patterns (PAMPs)(Uematsu & Akira, 2006). Further, PRR-induced ligand binding triggers internal signaling cascades that result in nucleus-based gene expression. Innate immune cells produce cytokines, chemokines, and antimicrobial agents, which, in turn, activate effector cells, attract them to the infection site, and eradicate infections, respectively. The main fungal PAMPs that the host innate immune system can identify are found in the cell wall.

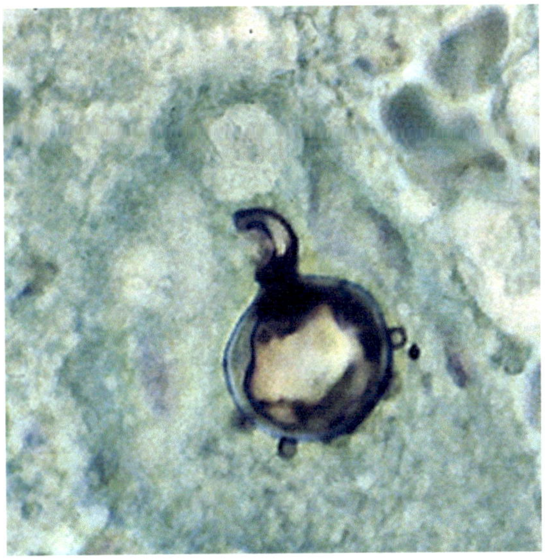

Figure 5.8 *Paracoccidioides brasiliensis*

Source: https://upload.wikimedia.org/wikipedia/commons/8/8c/Paracoccidioides_brasiliensis_tissue_GMS.jpg,*Creative Commons License.*

β-1,3-glucan is one of the powerful fungal PAMPs, and it is typically covered by other carbohydrates. In many pathogenic fungi, the sequestration of β-1,3-glucan by less immunostimulatory cell wall components has developed into a powerful immune evasion approach or strategy. Examples of this include the rodlet layer of airborne fungal spores, like Aspergillus species, the masking of β-glucans by mannans in Candida species, the presence of α-glucans in the outer cell wall of Histoplasma and *Paracoccidioides brasiliensis* (Figure 5.8), and the capsule enclosing *Cryptococcus neoformans*. Therefore, β-1,3-glucan exposure increases immunogenicity. This occurs during the infection process when the fungal cell wall's natural integrity and architecture are disrupted by antifungal medications like echinocandins or host-derived lytic enzymes that attack the cell wall. The dynamics of the fungal cell wall in response to environmental stimuli also expose β-1,3-glucans specifically in *C. albicans* and *A. fumigatus*(Childers et al., 2020). The primary PRRs implicated in fungus recognition are members of the myeloid C-type lectin receptor (CLR) family, which is extensively expressed by macrophages, neutrophils, and dendritic cells (DCs). One or more C-type lectin-like domains (CTLDs), many of which bind to carbohydrates like those in the fungal cell wall, are what distinguish CLRs from one another. The family of CLRs includes endocytic receptors that internalize their ligands, like the mannose receptor (MR), signaling receptors that function as PRRs to start innate and adaptive immunity, soluble molecules that activate the complement cascade, like the mannose-binding protein (MBP) or surfactant protein D, and others that have immunomodulatory properties. Dectin-1 is the prototypic signaling CLR. It attaches itself to the fungal cell wall β-(1,3)-glucans. In its cytoplasmic domain, Dectin-1 has an ITAM-like motif known as hemITAM. The spleen tyrosine kinase (Syk) is recruited when Src-family kinases dimerize and phosphorylate a tyrosine residue of this motif. This tyrosine kinase then couples to the canonical NF-κB pathway through the adaptor protein CARD9 and the protein kinase C δ (PKCδ)(Chen & Gao, 2024). Dectin-1-mediated selective signaling is qualitatively different from TLR-mediated signaling because it induces significant amounts of TNF, IL-6, and IL-23 but low IL-12. The phospholipase Cγ2-dependent nuclear factor of activated T cell (NFAT) activation can be triggered by dectin-1 signaling, which will produce IL-2 and IL-10. Dectin-1 signaling triggers caspase-1 activation, which cleaves pro-IL-1β into mature IL-1β, resulting in the induction of IL-1β. Dectin-1 is primarily produced by myeloid immune cells, but it has also been shown to be expressed on epithelial cells and exhibit Syk-dependent pro-inflammatory cytokine production in response to pure β-glucans and fungal cells.

5.10 Animal model studies

In animal models involving C. albicans, *A. fumigatus*, and Pneumocystis, among other dangerous fungi, dectin-1 signaling was shown to have a host-protective function. Dectin-1 polymorphisms have been linked in humans to increased vulnerability to invasive pulmonary aspergillosis as well as vulvovaginal candidiasis and onychomycosis. More research is necessary to determine the exact function of dectin-1 in defense against many human diseases. The Y238X polymorphism in dectin-1 is highly prevalent in the human population, raising doubts about its association with the disease(Gnat et al., 2021). Two more Syk-coupled CLRs that can identify fungal α-mannan structures are dectin-2 and mincle. They do not have the hemiTAM motif in their cytoplasmic tail like dectin-1 does. Rather, they come together using FcRγ, a signaling adapter that contains ITAM. It has recently been demonstrated that dectin-2 and mincle interact with MCL to improve ligand binding. Immunity against *Candida albicans*, *Candida glabrata*, and *Malassezia* is enhanced by dectin-2 signaling. The preferential binding of mincle to *Malassezia* spp. among fungal species, studies indicate that mincle agonists appear to be more limited among fungal pathogens than the wide range of fungi activating dectin-2. It has been demonstrated more recently that mincle plays a role in detecting *F. pedrosoi*, the cause of chromoblastosis, and it may also be able to identify Candida albicans. The mincles in mycobacteria have a ligand and react to a self-ligand released by dying cells. Deficits in Card9, a signaling component shared by all myeloid signaling CLR pathways, result in more severe problems in the regulation of fungal infections, whereas errors in specific CLRs can cause partial and/or selective defects in antifungal defense. Similarly, human persistent and severe fungal infections that mainly affect the skin and subcutaneous tissue, mucosal surfaces, and/or the central nervous system are linked to CARD9 polymorphisms. Instead of using an ITAM domain, many fungal CLRs were shown to communicate through an immunoreceptor tyrosine-based inhibitory motif (ITIM). ITIM phosphorylation and the interaction of SH2 domain-containing protein tyrosine phosphatases (SHP-1 and SHP-2) are the outcomes of ligand binding to ITIM-containing receptors. These tyrosine phosphatases then have regulatory effects on other activation pathways.

5.11 Receptors

The mannose receptor (MR), the first mannan-binding receptor identified, uses eight extracellular CTLDs to identify a variety of fungi and other microorganisms(Gupta & Gupta, 2012). It is possible to release soluble MR with retained ligand binding ability by cleaving the extracellular domain of the MR. The absence of a known signaling motif in its cytoplasmic tail indicates that the MR may instead function as a binding coreceptor to improve the function of signal receptors, even though it was demonstrated to boost ROS and cytokine production. Some TLRs, including TLR2, TLR4, TLR7, and TLR9, are also linked to fungus detection in addition to CLRs. TLRs are membrane-bound receptors made up of a conserved Toll/IL-1R-domain in the cytoplasmic domain and leucine-rich repeats for ligand binding. The latter facilitates signaling through MyD88, which couples to the stimulation of pro-inflammatory target genes and NF-κB activation. Fungal phospholipomannan and O-mannan structures are recognized by TLR2 and TLR4, which are expressed at the cell surface. In response to *Candida neoformans*, *A. fumigatus*, and *Candida albicans*, the endosomal TLRs TLR7 and TLR9 have also been linked to fungal recognition. In response to fungal stimuli, the TLR and CLR pathways interact, sometimes in a synergistic or antagonistic way. When dectin-1 and TLR2 are co-stimulated, the two pathways produce more TNF, IL-6, and IL-23(Dzopalic et al., 2012). Compared to TLR activation alone, the synergy between dectin-1 and TLR2 also modifies the overall cytokine response quality by shifting the relative amounts of IL-23 against IL-1. Further, TLR2 and SIGNR1 pathways also interact, but the results are different because SIGNR1 inhibits TLR2 activity and reduces the TLR2-induced response. TLRs and CLRs are not the only PRR pathways that cross-talk with one another. It has also been reported that various receptors from other PRR families can activate synergistically. The balanced activation of several PRRs is necessary for the generation of protective immunity against fungal infections.

5.12 Infections and cytokines

In addition to other cytokines and chemokines, IL-1β is produced by a variety of fungal infections. The production of bioactive IL-1β necessitates two separate signals. The first controls pro-IL-1β transcription and translation, while the second causes pro-IL-1β to be proteolytically cleaved into active IL-1β. Both stages of IL-1β production are initiated by fungi. They cause caspase-1 to cleave proteins by assembling inflammasomes with different subunit compositions. To provide a framework for caspase-1 activation, *Candida albicans* promotes the formation of an inflammasome made up of the NOD-like receptor NLRP3 and ASC. Mice lacking NLRP3 showed vulnerability to both superficial and systemic candidiasis, indicating the significance of the NLRP3 inflammasome in antifungal immunity. The yeast-to-hyphal transition is necessary for *C. albicans* to activate the NLRP3 inflammasome, which may be related to the fungal cell surface β-glucan exposure and the release of secreted aspartyl proteinase (SAP)2 and SAP6. Human monocytes infected with *A. fumigatus* also showed similar results. In a model of mixed candidiasis, it was demonstrated that the NLRC4 inflammasome, in addition to the NLRP3 inflammasome, promoted protective immunity against *Candida albicans*(Wellington et al., 2014). Enzymes other than caspase-1 can, at least in certain situations, process IL-1β. It was demonstrated that in response to Candida albicans, caspase-8, and ASC can be combined into a complex with CARD9/Bcl-10/MALT1 to create a noncanonical inflammasome that can process pro-IL-1β without the assistance of caspase-1. It might alter the NLRP3 inflammasome activity.

The fungal internalization did not affect *C. albicans* ability to assemble and activate the noncanonical caspase-8 inflammasome, suggesting that cytosolic NLRs are not necessary for this process. It has been proposed that the synthesis of IL-1β in some cell types occurs entirely independently of inflammasome activation. Human monocytes can emit bioactive IL-1β following stimulation by TLR2 or TLR4 alone or by stimulating TLR2, MR, and dectin-1 simultaneously. This is because human monocytes constitutively express caspase-1 and release ATP. Aspartyl proteases generated from *Candida albicans* and neutrophil-derived proteinase-3 can both process IL-1β. Nonclassical protein secretion, which is ER/Golgi independent and still poorly understood, is how the cell releases mature IL-1β. Since they both use the same receptor to signal, IL-1β and IL-1α are closely related. Although it is not a caspase-1 substrate, IL-1α still requires processing to become bioactive. However, by accelerating the processing of IL-1β, which was thought to bind to intracellular IL-1a and act as a vehicle for IL-1α release, the NLRP3 inflammasome and caspase-1 were indirectly linked to the secretion of IL-1α. Calpain I and II can cleave cell surface-bound IL-1α at the cell membrane, while extracellular proteases can process released pro-IL-1α. Cytolytic cell death also results in the release of IL-1α, which is constitutively produced in certain cells like keratinocytes.

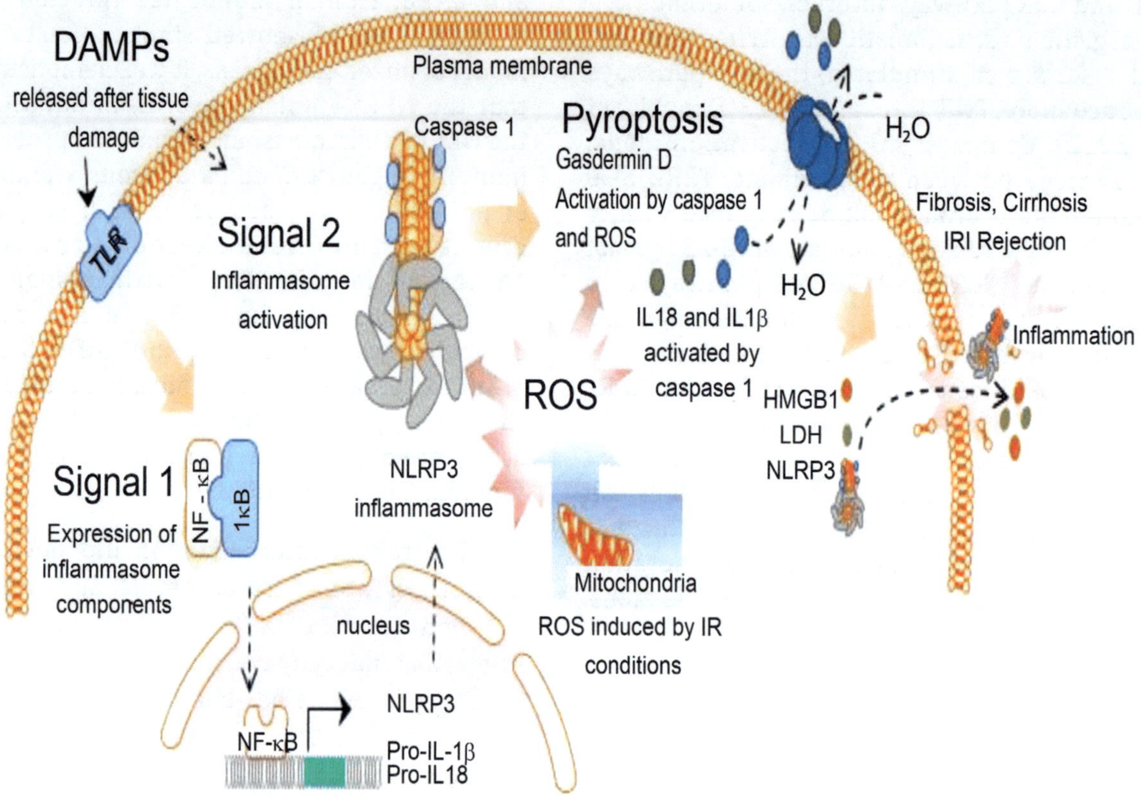

Figure 5.9 Pyroptosis

Source: Lucas-Ruiz, F., Peñín-Franch, A., Pons, J. A., Ramírez, P., Pelegrín, P., Cuevas, S., & Baroja-Mazo, A. (2022). Emerging Role of NLRP3 Inflammasome and Pyroptosis in Liver Transplantation. International Journal of Molecular Sciences, 23(22), 14396. https://doi.org/10.3390/ijms232214396,*Creative Commons License.*

5.13 Pyroptosis

Activation of caspase-1 can also cause pyroptosis, (Figure 5.9) an inflammatory kind of programmed cell death, in addition to its crucial role in processing IL-1β(Kesavardhana et al., 2020). Chromatin condensation and DNA fragmentation are the outcomes of pyroptosis. However, pyroptosis involves cell swelling, pore-mediated lysis, and the release of intracellular components such as cytoplasmic cytokines like IL-1α and IL-1β ATP, high mobility group box 1 (HMGB1), and nucleic acids that are typically not exposed to the extracellular compartment, in contrast to apoptosis, which is a non-lytic mechanism. These molecules were also known as damage-associated molecular patterns (DAMPs) because of their propensity to cause inflammation when released into the extracellular environment. Cellular receptors that stimulate inflammatory responses have been found for a few of them. Thus, caspase-1 activation is a crucial host mechanism for assessing the level of risk posed by a specific infection. A key factor in bloodstream infections is complement activation. Fungal infections quickly activate the complement through a variety of mechanisms, such as the alternative complement pathway, which has been demonstrated for both Zygomycetes and *Candida albicans*. Fast C3 convertase activation causes *C. albicans* opsonization through C3b binding to β-(1,6)-glucan, which enables neutrophil phagocytosis in a CR3-dependent manner(Speth et al., 2007). The complement activation also causes anaphylatoxins C3a and C5a to be produced, which have significant immunostimulatory effects, especially on neutrophils and monocytes, which are prevalent in the bloodstream and can serve as chemoattractants for these cells in tissues. Mice deficient in either C3 or C5 have vulnerability to systemic candidiasis. An abnormal inflammatory response, characterized by an enhanced production of TNF and IL-6, is linked to the higher susceptibility in cases with C5 deficiency. In response to Candida albicans, C5a increases the production of cytokines from human PBMCs. Therefore, rapid complement activation is essential for acute antifungal defense, particularly in cases of fungemia.

5.14 Immune reactions

Fungal pathogens come into contact with various immune cells within the tissue; some of these cells live constitutively in peripheral tissue during homeostasis, while others only enter the tissue when an infection occurs. In recent years, there has been a growing interest in tissue-resident (TR) immune cells. Many myeloid and lymphoid TR cell subgroups were found. Their distribution is highly tissue-dependent; some are restricted to the central nervous system, the skin epidermis, or the lung alveolar region. Myeloid cells found in bone marrow, blood, and secondary lymphoid organs are ontogenically different from myeloid TR cells. They self-renew from local precursors and are seeded as early as embryonic hematopoiesis. This is less evident for lymphoid-lineage TR cells. TR immune cells are positioned carefully to respond quickly to invasive pathogens and to protect the skin and mucosa. Alveolar macrophages, which dwell in the airways, play a key role in host defense against airborne infections. Inhaled fungal spores, such as those of *A. fumigatus*, are generally taken up and destroyed efficiently by alveolar macrophages. Fungal absorption was demonstrated to be promoted by pentraxin-3. Oxidative mechanisms in alveolar macrophages are responsible for restricting germination and killing the phagocytosed *A. fumigatus* spores. However, if this process is not successful, the infection can develop toward invasive pulmonary aspergillosis. During systemic candidiasis, CX3CR1+ macrophages in the kidney are necessary for very early renal control of the fungus. Mice with CX3CR1 loss have impaired protection against infection, which impacts the survival of TR macrophages. Although the relationship between these cells and TR macrophages is still unclear, the interaction of macrophages with fungal infections has been thoroughly investigated in vitro utilizing macrophage cell lines, macrophages generated from human blood monocytes, and macrophages derived from murine bone marrow progenitors. Following phagocyte absorption, fungal infections have been found to employ a variety of survival strategies. In fact, *C. neoformans* can live and multiply inside the phagosomes of macrophages. By preventing phagolysosomal fusion and changing the phagolysosomal pH, *H. capsulatum*, *C. glabrata*, and *C. albicans* can prevent phagosomal maturation. *Candida albicans* and *A. fumigatus* can interfere with the phagosome and evade macrophages; this frequently results in host cell death. NADPH oxidase inhibits *C. albicans* filamentation inside macrophages in vivo, as demonstrated by imaging of C. albicans-macrophage interactions in a zebrafish model(Sonnberger et al., 2024). In addition to ROS-mediated strategies, macrophages have evolved supplementary tactics to counteract fungal development within the phagolysosome. The change in metal homeostasis brought on by cytokines during *Histoplasma capsulatum* infection serves as an example this. To inhibit fungal replication and encourage fungal clearance, GM-CSF causes the phagolysosome to selectively shift zinc ions to the Golgi.

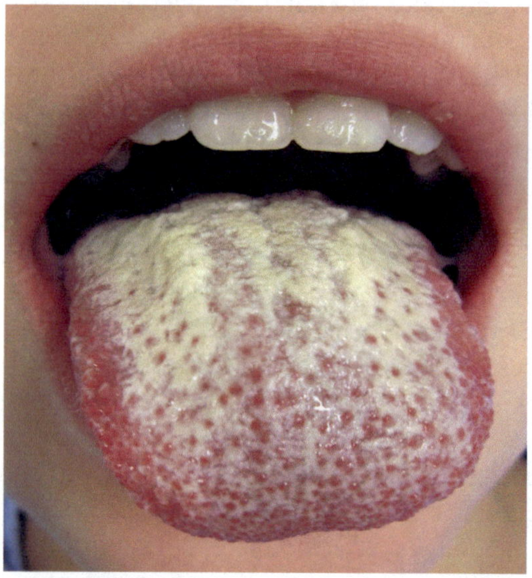

Figure 5.10 Systemic candidiasis

Source: https://upload.wikimedia.org/wikipedia/commons/a/a0/Human_tongue_infected_with_oral_candidiasis.jpg,*Creative Commons License.*

Apart from myeloid TR cells, TR lymphocytes with tissue-specific distribution and function, such as γδ T cells and RAG-independent innate lymphoid cells, are also present in the skin and mucosa. One thing they have in common with ordinary T cells is that they are programmed to create cytokines in response to inflammatory or infectious stimuli. However, the kinetics of cytokine production are significantly faster. Innate lymphocytes are involved in maintaining the balance of commensal microbiota in barrier tissues in addition to their defense against infections. If dysregulated, they may also exacerbate autoimmune and autoinflammatory diseases. Innate lymphocyte ability to produce IL-17 in mice with superficial candidiasis was the primary focus of research on fungal infections. The most prevalent leukocytes in circulation, neutrophils typically serve as the first line of defense against invasive microorganisms. The correlation between fungal infections and neutropenia demonstrates their critical involvement in antifungal immunity.

Systemic candidiasis (Figure 5.10) is a common side effect of leukemia patients receiving neutrophil-depleting cytotoxic treatment(Teoh & Pavelka, 2016). Similarly, deficiencies in neutrophil functions, such as leukocyte adhesion deficiency (LAG), increase the risk of *Pneumocystis carinii* infections, invasive pulmonary aspergillosis is linked to NADPH oxidase deficiency, and MPO-deficient people have a higher risk of *C. albicans* infections. It is yet unknown why and how distinct neutrophil abnormalities are linked to various disease types, even though these instances amply demonstrate the critical role neutrophils play in systemic fungal infections. Neutrophils are primarily found in the blood to offer defense against blood-borne pathogens, but they are also found in the tissues in low concentrations and are quickly drawn in during infection and inflammation. Many compounds, including HDPs, anaphylatoxins, and CXC chemokines, exhibit chemotactic action toward neutrophils and many of them also support neutrophil function. Through both oxidative and nonoxidative processes, neutrophils exhibit a range of antibacterial activity against both intracellular and external microorganisms. Yeast cells and fungal spores are among the microorganisms that neutrophils effectively absorb. Following internalization, the phagosome matures and the NADPH oxidase complex is assembled at the phagosomal membrane. Non-ingestible particles can also cause the NADPH oxidase complex to develop at the plasma membrane.

5.15 Respiratory problems

The respiratory burst is the term used to describe the production of superoxide, which is dependent on NADPH, and the subsequent production of reactive oxygen species (ROS) (Thomas, 2017). Because of their strong fungicidal potential, ROS are an essential part of the antimicrobial defense against both intracellular and extracellular fungi. The respiratory burst further aids in the destruction of microorganisms by triggering a potassium influx and activating antifungal proteases inside the phagosome. The neutrophil oxidative mechanism is the inducible nitric oxide synthase (iNOS), which produces reactive nitrogen intermediates. Its applicability to antifungal defense is uncertain, and data from studies using animals without iNOS indicates that it might be necessary for the management of a small number of specific infections, including *C. neoformans*. The granules containing proteases and other antimicrobial effectors are carried by neutrophils. As neutrophils mature in the bone marrow, distinct subsets of granules are generated. Certain granules are rich in lactoferrin and lysozyme, whereas tertiary granules, also known as gelatinase granules, include gelatinase and matrix metalloprotease (MMP9). Azurophilic granules contain myelopreoxidase (MPO), cathepsin G, neutrophil elastase, proteinase 3, and other substances. Neutrophil-produced host defense peptides (HDPs) like cathelicidins and α-defensins are stored in neutrophil granules. When the granules fuse with the phagosome, the microbes are exposed to these proteases and antimicrobials. To release the granule content in the extracellular space against extracellular microorganisms, granules also fuse with the plasma membrane in a process known as degranulation. It was shown that granule proteases, specifically cathepsin G and neutrophil elastase, are important for killing fungi. The neutrophils release cytokines that enhance their own antifungal properties and aid in the overall control of the immune response. The primary source of IL-17 during fungal keratitis is neutrophils rather than lymphoid-lineage cells.

5.16 The NETosis defense mechanism

The process of NETosis is the neutrophil-mediated defensive mechanism(Lehman & Segal, 2020). Neutrophils can discharge DNA with microbicidal proteins attached, which can serve as extracellular traps for microbes. It has been demonstrated that fungal hyphae, which are large to be phagocytosed, but not yeast cells, selectively trigger this process, which is also thought to be an alternate method of neutrophil cell death. Chromatin decondensation, granule and nuclear envelope membrane disintegration, and cell membrane disruption are all components of NETosis. This depends on the enzyme peptidyl arginine deiminase type IV (PAD4), which alters histone arginine residues to encourage chromatin decondensation, as well as NADPH oxidase and MPO. Restoring NADPH shortage in CGD patients with gene therapy alleviated NET formation and reduced the patient's vulnerability to *A. nidulans*. Granule proteases and cytoplasmic effector proteins like calprotectin are used to decorate NETs. NETs may serve as a scaffold for fungicidal (fungistatic) functions in addition to offering a physical trap for pathogens. Therefore, NETosis might be an adaptation to infection by pathogens. Blood-derived monocytes also aid in host defense, even though neutrophils are the main inflammatory effector cells against fungal infections. A mouse model of invasive pulmonary aspergillosis was used for the research. Innate defense against *A. fumigatus* is facilitated by CCR^{2+} inflammatory monocytes in different ways. Monocytes are necessary for the synthesis of IL-1α, which stimulates the production of chemokines and the recruitment of neutrophils, and modifies the lung inflammation to increase neutrophil candidacidal activity. The inflammatory monocytes provide protection when systemic candidiasis is present. Due to their ability to develop into DCs and/or macrophages in inflammatory environments, inflammatory monocytes also aid in the host's defense against fungal infection. TR macrophages and monocyte-derived macrophages are believed to behave similarly. However, by priming $CD4^+$ T cells, monocyte-derived DCs support adaptive immunity against *A. fumigatus*, and *B. dermatitidis*(Loh & Lam, 2023). Training monocytes is linked to epigenetic reprogramming in response to β-glucans in fungal and *Candida albicans* cell walls, which causes a change in metabolism reliant on the activation of hypoxia-inducible factor-1α (HIF-1α) and mammalian target of rapamycin (mTOR).

5.17 NK cells

NK cells are members of the ILC family. Because of their ability to kill target cells through perforin and death ligand-mediated pathways, NK cells are also referred to as killing ILCs to differentiate them from the family of helper ILCs. Although NK cells are only sporadically distributed across tissues in a stable state, they can be drawn into organs in response to inflammatory situations. NK cell ability to combat a variety of fungal infections was initially evaluated in vitro.

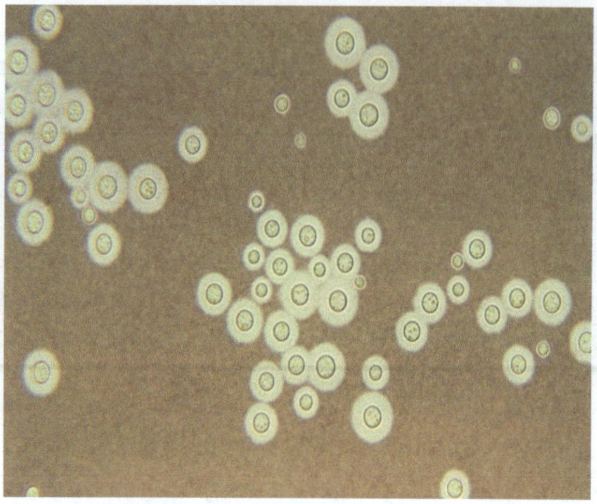

Figure 5.11 *Cryptococcus neoformans*

Source: https://upload.wikimedia.org/wikipedia/commons/6/6f/Cryptococcus_neoformans_using_a_light_India_ink_staining_preparation_PHIL_3771_lores.jpg,*Creative Commons License.*

It was discovered that NK cells killed the hyphal form of *A. fumigatus*, *Cryptococcus neoformans* (Figure 5.11), and Mucormycetes. It has been demonstrated that mouse-derived NK cells have antifungal activity against *Candida albicans*, whereas human NK cells have no antifungal activity against the same fungus. NK cells can kill pathogens directly as well as via secreting cytokines, specifically TNF, and GM-CSF, which can improve neutrophil and macrophage survival and antimicrobial activity. In fact, it was demonstrated that cytokines from NK cells induced by *Candida albicans* could increase neutrophil antifungal activity. NK cells can function as a supplier of IFN-γ during infection in vivo, which is necessary to protect neutropenic mice against *A. fumigatus*. In a mouse model (*C. neoformans*) infection, NK cells are also necessary for fungal control. By secreting GM-CSF, which is triggered by IL-23p19 produced from CD11c+ cells, NK cells also play a crucial part in systemic candidiasis. The generation of GM-CSF from NK cells in turn enhances neutrophil activity and survival. NK cells seem to have minimal effect on fungal defense in barrier tissues, such as during OPC, which is consistent with the original function in systemic immunity. NKT cells participate in host defense against *A. fumigatus* and have characteristics in common with both T cells and NK cells. Fungal lipids don't get involved in direct NKT cell activation, but DC identification of β-glucans and IL-12 synthesis stimulate NKT cells. This mechanism might be generally applicable to NKT cell responses to antifungals. The antimicrobial effector molecules, including ROS and proteases, can damage the host even though they were evolved for host protection. Therefore, strict control of inflammatory responses is necessary for their host benefit.

Neutrophil immunopathological roles during systemic candidiasis have also been reported. Prolonged neutrophil stay in the kidney is linked to immunopathology, whereas early neutrophil recruitment to the diseased organs is linked to fungal clearance. CCR1 is necessary for immunopathology and the recruitment of neutrophils to the kidney; its removal improves renal function and host survival(Ramos et al., 2012). As demonstrated in the systemic candidiasis in mice, where it induced an overt neutrophil response, IFN type I signaling can also be harmful to the host. Similarly, even while neutrophils exhibit fungicidal activity against this pathogen in vitro, they may increase vulnerability rather than protect from infection during pulmonary cryptococcosis. As demonstrated by the correlation between deficiencies in T cell immunity and serious fungal diseases such superficial candidiasis, histoplasmosis, and cryptococcal infections, adaptive immunity and CD4+ T cells in particular are essential for defense against many fungal infections.

5.18 T-cells and other molecules

Primary immunodeficiencies that affect T cell growth or function, such as severe combined immunodeficiency (SCID), and corticosteroid therapy are T cell abnormalities that expose us to fungal infections. For many years, research was conducted on the immune role ofT-cells against fungal infections. Because every T cell carries antigen receptors with a unique specificity, the whole T cell population exhibits an almost infinite variety of distinct antigenic specificities. Germline-encoded gene segments undergo somatic recombination to produce the T cell repertoire. Only peptide antigens presented in the presence of MHC class II molecules are recognized by CD4+ T lymphocytes. Naïve T cells must be stimulated by cognate antigen-MHC-II complexes presented by antigen-presenting cells to activate and expand clonally, which comes before they differentiate into effector T cells, to become completely functional. Although a complex microorganism, like a fungus, can theoretically produce an almost infinite range of antigenic peptides, T cell unique responses to a particular pathogen during infection are constrained to a small number of epitopes. Immunodominant T cell epitopes are a small number of unique peptides that frequently account for a large fraction of all pathogen-specific T cells.

Only a small number of fungal T-cell epitopes have been found. These include the pALS3236–253 and pADH126–140 epitopes, which are derived from *Candida albicans* and are functionally conserved in a variety of non-albicans species of the fungus. A substantial portion of all *C. albicans*-specific CD4+ T cells in mice and humans recognize pALS3236–253, which, if administered as a vaccine, offers defense against experimental *C. albicans* infection. Although the exact range of amino acids binding to MHC-II molecules has not been established, it has been demonstrated that many other fungal antigens, including the 65-kDa mannoprotein MP65 from *Candida albicans* and the heat shock protein from *H. capsulatum* and Paracoccidioides, function as T cell antigens(Gow et al., 2017). Fungal calnexin, which is typically found in the ER but can also be seen on the fungal cell surface, was recently discovered to be a novel T cell antigen that is shared by Ascomycota, which includes opportunistic molds, thermally dimorphic fungi, and *Pseudogymnoascus destructans*, the fungus that causes bats to develop white nose syndrome. Compared to control subjects, human T cells from people who had previously contracted a thermally dimorphic fungal infection showed a stronger reaction to calnexin. As antigen-presenting cells (APCs), dendritic cells (DCs) stimulate the activation and development of naïve T cells into effector and memory T cells. In response to microbial signals that promote antigen uptake, processing, and presentation, as well as increased production of costimulatory molecules and secretion of inflammatory cytokines, pattern recognition receptors (PRR) signaling controls the APC function of DCs. This coordinated process, also known as DC maturation, is necessary for effective T cell priming and is linked to the DC migration from the peripheral site of infection to the draining lymph node. The newly activated T cells polarize into distinct subgroups of effector cells, such as Th1, Th2, Th17, and regulatory T cells or Treg, based on the strength of the signals generated by the APCs, which is determined by the combination of PRRs triggered. TGF-β and IL-6 encourage $CD4^+$ T cells to differentiate into Th17 cells, while IL-12 encourages them to differentiate into Th1 cells. IL-23 is necessary for Th17 maintenance. With Th1 cells secreting IFN-γ and Th17 cells secreting IL-17, each fraction of effector T cells generates a distinct set of effector cytokines. These cytokines activate unique effector responses that aid in pathogen removal but, in the event of dysregulation, may also encourage immunopathology. Thus, the induction of a specific innate signaling pathway in the APCs is linked to the activation of a specific effector response to a specific pathogen.

5.19 Other responses

The polarization of T-cell responses can be influenced by tissue-specific and environmental variables. In response to systemic infection, the oral mucosa produces a selective Th17 response, the skin produces a mixed but balanced Th17/Th1 response, and the body produces a dominant Th1 response with a negligible fraction of Th17 cells. Although the exact causes of these tissue-specific variations are unknown, it is believed that they result from variations in the DC composition of different tissues as well as the varying contributions of substances from other cells that can regulate the overall response. The development of Th17 responses also seems to be influenced by the presence of regulatory T cells, or Tregs(Lee et al., 2009). By ingesting IL-2, which can have Th17-inhibitory effects, they were demonstrated to encourage the development of Th17 cells in response to C. albicans. In response to fungal stimuli, Tregs themselves can transform into cells that produce IL-17. Tregs can therefore contribute to protective immunity against fungal infections in addition to their function in preserving tolerance and immunological homeostasis. Different subsets of mononuclear phagocytes (MNPs) are included in DCs. They constitutively dwell in secondary lymphoid organs or in peripheral tissue like the skin and mucosa, and they typically express high amounts of CD11c and MHC-II. Different developmental pathways give rise to DC subsets from precursors. Using a common DC progenitor (CDP) and a common macrophage and DC progenitor (MDP), DCs develop in a Flt3-dependent manner. They can be identified by functional differences and exist as either Batf3-dependent or Batf3-independent subgroups. Different T cell subsets seem to have the ability to selectively guard or protect against various disease types, which is consistent with the variable activation of T cell subsets during fungal infections. While Th17 cells are efficient against external bacteria and fungi in barrier tissues, Th1 cells are generally believed to defend against intracellular pathogens by enhancing phagocyte function. Th17 cells have drawn a lot of interest in recent years due to their nonredundant function in preventing superficial candidiasis. This might be especially important in situations where there is a CD4 deficiency, like in HIV/AIDS patients. In the absence of $CD4^+$ T cells, $CD8^+$ T cells can offer protection and stop fungal overgrowth. Innate lymphocytes have become significant substitute sources of IL-17. Their protective function was demonstrated in mice with OPC and cutaneous candidiasis.

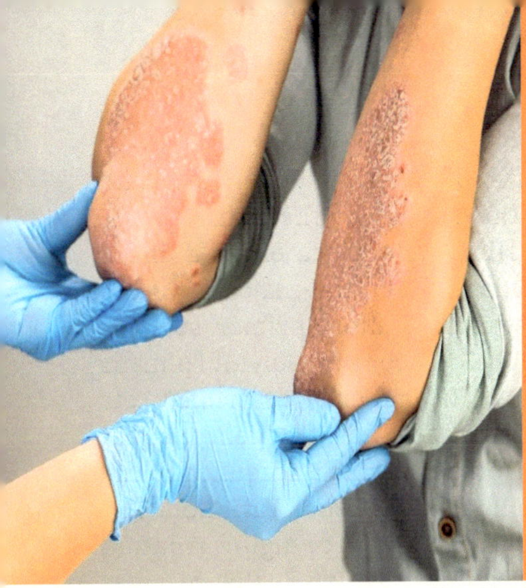

Chapter 6

CLINICAL PRACTICE AND IMMUNOGENETICS

Contents

6.1 Introduction

Olerup and Zetterquist were the first to develop HLA-SSP typing of the HLA-DR genes(Dunckley, 2012). Sequence-specific primer (SSP) typing of additional human leukocyte antigen (HLA) (Figure 6.1) class I and II genes was made possible by following technical advancements.

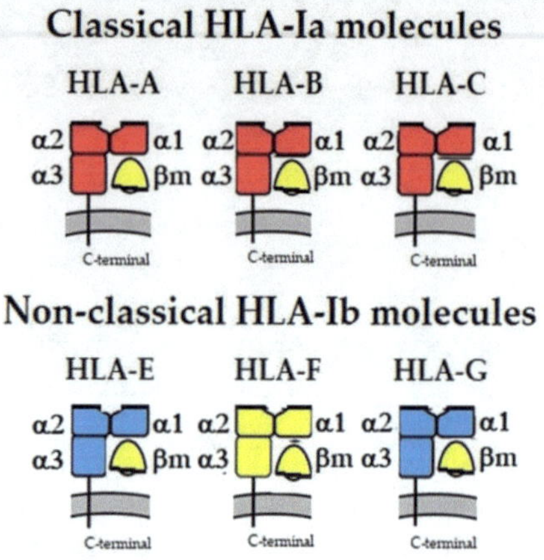

Figure 6.1 Human leukocyte antigen

Source: Ravindranath MH, Ravindranath NM, Selvan SR, Hilali FE, Amato-Menker CJ, Filippone EJ. Cell Surface B2m-Free Human Leukocyte Antigen (HLA) Monomers and Dimers: Are They Neo-HLA Class and Proto-HLA? Biomolecules. 2023; 13(8):1178. https://doi.org/10.3390/biom13081178,*Creative Commons License.*

6.2 Genotyping HLA alleles

For the HLA-(A to C), DRB1, DRB(3-5), and DQB1 alleles, Researchers created a thorough SSP typing system in 1995. All of the PCRs in this system were made to function under the same thermocycler conditions. Primers complementary to specific HLA allele sequences or a collection of related alleles are used in SSP typing. Primers are made so that the polymorphism that has to be found is at the 3' end. Taq DNA polymerase will not extend the primer if the 3' end of the primer does not match the HLA allele. Since exons 2 and 3 of the class I genes cover the majority of the known polymorphisms, most primer sets for HLA-(A to C) typing identify polymorphisms in these regions. The majority of primer sets for the HLA-DR, -DQ, and -DP genes cover exon 2 polymorphisms, which account for the majority of the known sequence variation. The SSP approach can be applied to high-resolution typing or low-resolution typing, which resolves alleles to the antigenic level. Primers are prepared first, distributed into PCR tubes or microtiter trays, and frozen for use in HLA-SSP typing. The primer sets can be kept between 2°C and 8°C if they are freeze-dried. When a person needs HLA genotyping, DNA is extracted, typically from a blood sample, and put into a buffer that has already been prepared with dNTPs and Taq DNA polymerase. The mixture is then aliquoted into microtiter plates with the primer sets, which are then put through the PCR procedure. By electrophoresing the PCR products across an agarose gel containing a dye that binds to DNA, like ethidium bromide, amplification is observed. The presence or lack of amplified HLA alleles can be seen when the gel is exposed to ultraviolet light.

As new HLA alleles were found, laboratories had to buy primers, set up their own SSP type trays, and keep their methods up-to-date during the early years of SSP technique development. However, the technology was quickly brought to market, and as a result, SSP typing kits for typing the HLA class I and II loci at either low or high resolution have been available. This just requires the lab to extract DNA from clinical samples, mix DNA and Taq DNA polymerase using pre-made buffer and primer sets that are sold commercially, run PCR, then run gels to see the amplification. Commercial HLA-SSP kit vendors also have software to help with result interpretation and HLA genotyping, although product assignment necessitates the usage of customized software due to the constantly growing number of HLA alleles. The main benefit of the SSP approach is that it is a very quick way of genotyping HLA; the entire procedure, including DNA extraction, takes two to three hours to complete. As a result, the method works well for genotyping organ transplant donors or urgent situations like patients in need of HLA-matched platelet transfusions. Even with the use of robotics or multi-dispensing pipettes, the SSP approach is not appropriate for typing large quantities of samples due to the number of PCRs needed for each sample, which must also be taken into account. There are commercial kits that use 96 PCRs per sample to conduct low-resolution HLA-A, B, and DRB1 typing(Williams et al., 2004). Resolving the major allele groups using a one-step SSP procedure is getting harder due to the continuously growing number of HLA alleles. Newly discovered alleles can be included by adding more primer mixes.

6.3 HLA-SSO typing

One of the earliest PCR-based HLA typing techniques was HLA-SSO typing, which was first created for the HLA class II loci and subsequently for the HLA class I genes. The method entails first extracting DNA, and then amplifying a specific HLA gene region, such as HLA-A, HLA-B, or HLA-DRB1. In a single PCR tube, primers are chosen to amplify every known allele of the specific HLA locus that has to be genotyped. Since these are the gene sections or fragments with the majority of the known sequence variation, exons 2 and 3 are often co-amplified as a single PCR product for HLA class I type, whereas only exon 2 is amplified for HLA class II typing. A positively charged nylon membrane is used to blot the amplified DNA, allowing the negatively charged DNA to adhere firmly. The size of the membrane can be raised as the quantity of samples increases, and many samples can be blotted onto the same membrane. Each oligonucleotide probe used in the genotyping process has its own membrane made using the amplified DNA samples. The membrane holding the attached DNA is put in a container and combined with a hybridization solution that contains an oligonucleotide that has a DNA sequence specific to a given HLA allele or set of alleles and is labeled with a marker like biotin. Hybridization happens when the amplifiable DNA sequence complements the oligonucleotide sequence. Like other oligonucleotides that are not specifically attached to the amplified DNA on the nylon membrane, non-hybridized oligonucleotides stay unbound in the solution and are readily eliminated in a series of rigorous washing procedures. Oligonucleotides are made so that the polymorphism to be detected is in the middle of the oligonucleotide sequence to promote the possible interaction between the oligonucleotide and the amplified DNA. Only one portion of the oligonucleotide binds to the amplified DNA if there is a sequence variation between the amplicon and the end of the oligonucleotide, increasing the possibility that it will wash off during the washing step. The presence of bound oligonucleotides can be detected by a chemiluminescent reaction. Each sample response to each oligonucleotide is noted, and the pattern of positive reactions allows for the assignment of the sample HLA type.

6.4 Sequencing

Large sample numbers can be easily typed using the sequence-specific oligonucleotide (SSO) method; for example, a standard typing lab with one or two 96-well microtiter trays can test 88-184 samples in a single assay. Because the SSO technique does not differentiate between cis and trans polymorphisms, it is unable to resolve all ambiguities due to the extremely large number of potential heterozygous HLA allele combinations. SSP typing, on the other hand, helps to resolve certain ambiguities by identifying alleles that share both the forward and reverse primer sequences on the same HLA allele, thereby connecting two polymorphic regions to the same allele. Although SSO typing is not a quick typing method, it takes around two days from the PCR stage to result assignment, it is a cost-effective method because one staff member can readily type 88-184 samples for a single gene locus in this time. The primers used in SSO typing are chosen from a non-variable region of the gene since they are made to amplify every allele for a certain locus. In general, the SSO approach is better than the SSP method at detecting new HLA alleles because a new allele will be amplified if it does not have a polymorphism in this region. A new allele should be identified that deviates from the typical patterns of known alleles if it possesses a polymorphism in one of the locations covered by an SSO. However, as the SSOs do not cover every area of the gene, novel alleles might still be ignored by this approach and would only be discovered if the material was genotyped using another technique, like DNA sequencing. Reverse-SSO is a method that works well for evaluating single samples or several samples at once, but the PCR-SSO approach is not a good methodology for small sample sizes. The reverse-SSO technique involves binding oligonucleotides one at a time to membranes, each of which has all the SSOs necessary for a certain HLA locus or allele group linked to it. Using primers designed specifically for the HLA locus to be typed, sample DNA is amplified and labeled with biotin(Erlich, 2012). After that, the pre-bound oligonucleotides hybridize with the amplified DNA to the membrane.

Washing eliminates non-specifically bound amplicons, and a chemiluminescent or color-based detection device is used to find the hybridization between the amplicon and membrane-bound oligonucleotide. The reverse-SSO system has a new version that uses Luminex xMAP technology (Trajanoski & Fidler, 2012).

6.5 Luminex xMAP technology

Polystyrene microspheres stained internally with red and infrared fluorophores are used in the Luminex xMAP technology (Figure 6.2). One hundred distinct sets of microspheres can be created by combining the two dyes in varying amounts on various beads. Even within the same reaction tube, each of the 100 bead sets may be uniquely identified using a Luminex analyzer. Every set of microspheres is coated with a distinct oligonucleotide for HLA genotyping. The procedure is performed in a 96-well PCR plate with one sample tested per well, enabling 96 samples to be evaluated concurrently. Test DNA is amplified by PCR and hybridized in solution. Washing removes non-hybridized DNA, and a fluorescent dye using a Luminex analyzer employing flow cytometric technology detects amplified DNA that has attached to the SSOs on the microspheres. In addition to providing quantitative results and HLA assignments, the analyzer automates the data collection process. A higher HLA typing resolution is made possible by Luminex xMAP technology, which makes it simpler to include more SSOs than other SSO or reverse-SSO techniques because each reaction tube or tray may hold 100 distinct bead sets. There are many commercial kits that use reverse-SSO typing, and although it still has the same ambiguity resolution issues as the original SSO method, it works well for genotyping tiny sample sizes. The approach can also be used for typing large sample quantities because some commercial kits use robotics for the hybridization, washing, and detection phases.

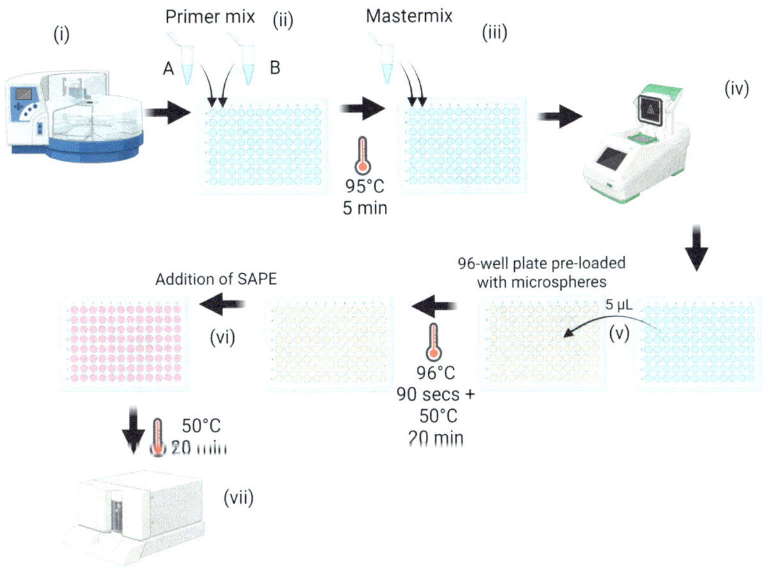

Figure 6.2 Luminex xMAP technology

Source: Ashby, M., Moore, R., King, S., Newbrook, K., Flannery, J., & Batten, C. (2024). Designing a Multiplex PCR-xMAP Assay for the Detection and Differentiation of African Horse Sickness Virus, Serotypes 1–9. Microorganisms, 12(5), 932. https://doi.org/10.3390/microorganisms12050932,*Creative Commons License.*

6.6 PCR approaches

Many techniques for HLA typing that use DNA amplification by the polymerase chain reaction (PCR) have been published. The ineffective PCR amplification of a primer with a 3' nucleotide mismatch is used in specific priming (SSP)(Sun et al., 2022). Because of this shortcoming, PCR primers that are specific for their target sequence can be created that won't amplify closely related sequences. A pattern of amplification corresponding to HLA alleles can be used to identify multiple nucleotide variations in HLA genes by standardizing the PCR cycle conditions for a variety of primers. Using fluorescently labeled dideoxynucleotides in a cycle sequencing reaction with a purified PCR result, SBT usually employs the Sanger technique. Precipitation or magnetic bead separation are used to clean the subsequent reaction of unincorporated dyes, dNTPs, and primers, and an automated analyzer detects the pieces that are left over. An automated analysis algorithm is used to analyze the nucleotide sequence from the fragment analysis and compare it to the known sequence of HLA alleles. Other methods involve applying next-generation sequencing or Sanger sequencing to sequence a single PCR result at each locus. Commercial software tools and the reagents for SSP and SBT for the majority of HLA loci are accessible. In a single well of a 96-well microtiter plate, immobilized biotinylated oligonucleotide probes are hybridized to PCR-amplified DNA using a series of microsphere beads in microbead hybridization tests. In a flow cytometric analysis device (Figure 6.3), fluorescent tagged PCR products positively hybridize with two internal fluorescent dyes to identify individual beads.

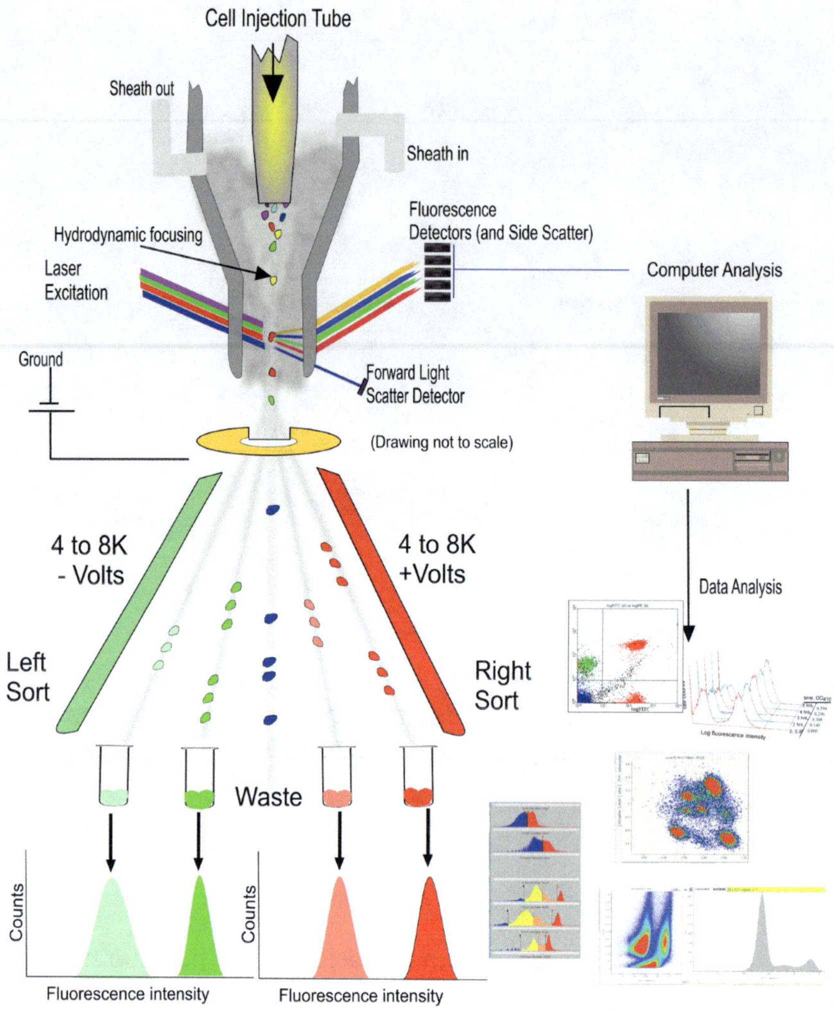

Figure 6.3 Flow cytometry

Source: Robinson, J. P., Ostafe, R., Iyengar, S. N., Rajwa, B., & Fischer, R. (2023). Flow Cytometry: The Next Revolution. Cells, 12(14), 1875. https://doi.org/10.3390/cells12141875,*Creative Commons License.*

Many solid-phase hybridization tests have been developed, such as the binding of an oligonucleotide probe or PCR product to a nylon membrane support and the detection of the probes by chemiluminescence. The PCR product is immobilized on a microtiter plate coated with streptavidin and hybridized with many fluorescent probes in a single microtiter plate well. The chelates of lanthanide metals that are used to label the probes have unique fluorescent properties that enable the identification of several probes in a single experiment. Typing single nucleotide polymorphisms (SNPs) that tag for HLA haplotypes is an alternate method of HLA genotyping. Only the related HLA-DQ2 and DQ8 haplotypes have six tagging SNPs for coeliac disease identified and confirmed in Caucasian populations. The approach is suitable for high-throughput screening assays and is cost-effective, but it is not advised for diagnostic testing since rare haplotypes make the specificities and sensitivities, which are high. The technique makes use of TaqMan chemistry and two allele-specific dual-labeled probes that bind to the SNP complementary target sequence in real-time PCR using alternate 5' dyes and a 3' quencher dye. The discrimination of alleles is made possible via positive hybridization, which releases a distinct reporter dye that can be detected by a fluorimeter. One high-resolution technique for identifying HLA polymorphisms is sequencing-based typing. Exons 2 and 3 can be used to distinguish the majority of HLA Class I alleles, while exon 2 is typically sufficient for Class II alleles. Depending on the clinical need and applicable requirements, additional sequencing may be necessary to rule out certain alleles with variations outside of exons 2 and 3 due to polymorphism sites in other exons. Target alleles are selectively amplified using PCR, the PCR products are then purified to eliminate excess primer and dNTPs, and the procedure concludes with agarose gel electrophoresis to evaluate the quantity and quality of the PCR products. After performing cycle sequencing reactions, the sequence reactions are purified before being electrophoresed using the Genetic Analyzer. Specialized software applications process the data and compare the sample sequence to the sequences of every theoretical allele combination to determine an accurate genotype.

6.7 Other techniques

Direct identification of new alleles is made possible by examining all nucleotides, both at conserved and polymorphic sites. This may not be achievable with methods like SSP and SSO typing. Commercial kits that contain primers for both PCR and sequencing for the majority of HLA loci are currently offered by several providers. As an alternative, a laboratory intending to use direct sequencing to achieve HLA typing can replicate several techniques. The ideal buffer conditions and heat cycling settings are then determined by optimizing the PCR conditions. The availability of sequence data is frequently the limiting barrier to such a strategy. A DNA template, a sequencing primer, thermally stable DNA polymerase, nucleotides (dNTPs), dideoxynucleotides (ddNTPs), in which each of the four dNTPs is labeled with one of the four specific fluorescent dyes, and buffer are needed for fluorescence-based cycle sequencing. A variety of extension products are produced and amplified by thermal cycling of the reactions, which stop when one of four fluorescently tagged dideoxynucleotides is added. The fluorescent dye on the extension product identifies the 3' terminal dideoxynucleotide as A, C, G, or T(Slatko et al., 1999). Each dye has a distinct wavelength that it produces when activated by a laser. In contrast to dye primer chemistry, dye terminator chemistry has the primary benefits of allowing the use of unlabeled sequencing primers, allowing the reactions to be carried out in a single tube, and requiring fewer pipetting steps. The polyacrylamide gels poured between two glass plates were used to segregate the results of DNA sequencing. Gel separation has been replaced by capillary electrophoresis employing a denaturing liquid polymer, which simplifies workflow, boosts throughput, and is simpler to use. The extension products of the sequencing procedure are injected into the capillary during capillary electrophoresis. The buffered sequence reaction is subjected to high voltage, which pushes the negatively charged fragments into the capillaries. Based on their overall cost, products are sorted by size. The fragments go via a laser beam on their way to the positive electrode, which causes the dyes to fluoresce. The signal is picked up by an optical detection device, and software transforms it into digital data.

The final sequence is then compared to a reference library to identify the allele combination present, and the data is analyzed using specialized software that aligns the resultant sequences and permits the operators to modify the base calls if necessary. Nowadays, DNA sequencing is a common high-throughput HLA-type method; tens of thousands of tests are performed annually by certain bone marrow donor registry typing institutions. By definition, DNA sequencing has the advantage of directly identifying every base in the DNA template. Sequence-specific PCR primers (PCR-SSP) and oligonucleotide probes (PCR-SSO) are examples of alternative molecular-based tests that only yield information for the areas to which the oligos are designed; no information is gained for the regions between primers and probes. Assign-SBT simplified the sequence analysis and allele assignment step of the test, whereas a single PCR per locus simplified the template production step. When combined, these advancements significantly simplified the SBT process and increased its cost-effectiveness. When combined, these advancements significantly simplified the SBT process and increased its cost-effectiveness. Assign-SBT was specifically created for routine high-throughput HLA typing. It included a special base caller made for precise base calling of heterozygous sequences as well as a special quality rating system that made it possible to identify low-quality sites in a sequence and, if they existed, base call errors with ease. The findings changed instantly after any alteration. The program was the first of its kind to offer a quantitative quality control system based on Shewhart analysis, allowing for quality assessment from sample to sample, run to run, and assay to assay. In addition to keeping up with the intricacies of HLA typing, Assign-SBT has developed further to give researchers the means to carry out further studies into HLA complexity and its connection to transplant biology and disease risk. At the feto-maternal interface, the non-classical human leukocyte antigen (HLA)-G is highly expressed; however, it is only weakly expressed in healthy tissues such as the thymus, cornea, erythroid cells, and blood cells(Buse & Markert, 2019). HLA-G is expressed in cancer, transplanted tissue, autoimmune disorders, and inflammation. This expression is always linked to the induction of tolerance through the suppression of innate and adaptive immune responses. HLA-G gene structure is similar to that of the traditional HLA class I genes: There are eight exons and seven introns in the HLA-G gene. Exon 5 represents the transmembrane region, exon 6 the cytoplasmic tail; exon 7 is never present in the mature mRNA; exon 8 is not translated due to an early stop codon in exon 6; and exon 1 encodes the peptide signal. Exons 2, 3, and 4 represent the extracellular domains, respectively. There is very little variation in HLA-G within the coding area. However, a longer polymorphism has been documented in the gene 3' untranslated region and 5' upstream regulatory region. 44 distinct HLA-G variants have been identified, according to the International Immunogenetics Database; 33 single nucleotide polymorphisms (SNPs) are located inside the HLA-G encoding region, and only 13 changes lead to an amino acid exchange. However, it must be noted that at least 24 of the 44 alleles exhibit a substitution.

The conformational alterations brought about by nucleotide mutations that cause amino acid shifts at the protein level may have an impact on biological activity. Only four of the thirty-three SNPs in the coding area of HLA-G are associated with an amino acid exchange, and these SNPs do exhibit frequencies above 1% in population studies concerning the allele HLA-G*01:01. One of them, which is common for the G*01:03 allele, is found at codon 31 in exon 2, where a threonine is substituted for a serine. In exon 3, two are located at codons 110 and 130. For the G*01:04 group, the first one leads to the amino acid exchange of leucine to isoleucine. The reading frame is altered and a stop signal (TGA) is produced in codon 189 at exon 4 when a cytosine at the first nucleotide of codon 130 in exon 3 is deleted. This genotype is known as the G*01:05N allele (N means null allele) because it lacks important information from the full-length transcript. The other SNPs are replacements that are synonymous. This gene segment is regarded as the 3' UTR of the mature RNA as exon 7 is missing from the mature mRNA and exon 8 is not translated because of the stop codon in exon 6. The HLA-G gene has a 14 bp fragment insertion/deletion (ins/del) polymorphism at 3' UTR. A 14 bp insertion in an HLA-G allele is linked to alternative splicing products that omit 92 bases from the 3' UTR(de Almeida et al., 2018). The 14 bp insertion itself is linked to decreased mRNA synthesis, even though such shortened mRNAs are said to be more stable. The promoter region now contains about 29 variation sites. The need for useful methods for the typing of the coding and non-coding regions of the HLA-G gene has been highlighted by the discovery that HLA-G significantly suppresses the immune system and that some HLA-G variations are linked to high and low expression levels that may be of functional relevance.

6.8 C4 immunogenetics

Genes at two loci in the major histocompatibility complex (MHC) on chromosome 6 code for the two C4 isotypes, C4A and C4B. The primary structural and functional differences between the C4 isotypes are caused by five nucleotide variations found in exon 26, although these isotypes share over 99% amino acid sequence identity. With more than 40 alleles, gene duplications, and null alleles, C4A and C4B are extremely polymorphic. Because of the presence or lack of an endogenous retroviral sequence, HERV-K(C4) in intron 9, the C4 genes can be either short (14.6 kb) or long (21 kb). For each haplotype, the C4 gene copy number (GCN) can range from 1 to 3, and for diploid genomes, it can range from 2 to 6. Healthy persons have a variety of C4 plasma protein concentrations due to variations in GCN. Those with short genes had comparatively greater C4 plasma levels than those with long genes, even when they had an identical number of C4 genes. Susceptibility to autoimmune disease may also result from variations in the C4 GCN, the gene size (long or short), and the C4 isotypes (C4A and C4B). So, a low blood C4 level in autoimmune disease patients may result from genetic causes or from continuous disease activity linked to complement activation and consumption. Making this distinction will have clinical ramifications. Because of the high degree of homology between C4A and C4B, it can be challenging to determine GCN precisely, but several methods have been developed. At least 26 constitutively and non-specifically expressed proteins make up the complement system. A series of processes must be triggered for these proteins to work. The complement cascade can be activated via various channels. Each of them is activated by various substances or methods. One route improves binding to CR1 and immune complex clearance, as well as preventing immune complex precipitation. Autoimmune diseases mediated by the immune complex are more likely to occur in individuals who are homozygous for the classical pathway C4, C2, and C1 components(Truedsson, 2015). Genes at two loci in the major histocompatibility complex (MHC) on chromosome 6 encode the C4 protein.

The presence or absence of a 6.5 kb endogenous retrovirus insertion, HERVK(C4) in intron 9 determines the length of each of these genes, resulting in long (22 kb) and short (14.6 kb) C4 genes. The products of these loci, C4A and C4B, share more than 99% of their amino acid sequences and show a very high degree of chromosomal sequence similarity across the C4 molecule. Even though the amino acids C4A and C4B are similar, they have different functions. While C4B preferentially attaches to acceptor hydroxyl groups that are mostly present on the carbohydrates of red blood cell surfaces, C4A preferentially binds to amino groups, such as those present in immune complexes. With more than 40 alleles, including null alleles and gene duplications, C4A and C4B are highly polymorphic. The lack of C4 protein in plasma defines C4 null alleles. They could result from mutations that cause non-expression, gene conversion, homo-duplication, or gene deletion. The range of C4 plasma protein concentrations is caused by variations in gene copy number (GCN). Reference ranges for blood C4 concentration were established. C4 protein level and activity appear to be influenced by the size of C4 genes; participants with short C4 genes showed higher C4 protein levels and higher C4 hemolytic activities than those with long genes alone. There have also been reports of a strong connection between the number of short genes with serum levels of C4B and the number of long genes with serum levels of C4A. 60.8% of individuals have four copies of the C4 gene, 27.2% have fewer than four copies, and 12% have more than four copies(Castley & Martinez, 2012). The GCN of C4 and surrounding genes can range from 1-3 per haplotype or 2-6 per diploid genome. A variety of genes, including the C4 genes, are carried by distinct ancestral haplotypes (AHs) of the MHC. It has been proposed that autoimmune disease susceptibility may result from variations in the C4 gene copy number, the polymorphism of gene size (long or short), and the C4 isotypes.

6.9 C4 amplification studies

The first report of a higher frequency of C4A null alleles in SLE was made in 1983. Many techniques, such as electrophoretic mobility of the entire protein or its subunits, serological analysis using the Rodgers (Rg) and Chido (Ch) determinant, and DNA-based techniques can be used to determine the polymorphism of C4. Because of the high degree of similarity between C4A and C4B, it can be challenging to determine GCN precisely. Only five nucleotide polymorphisms in exon 26 are responsible for the main structural and functional variations between the C4 isotypes, and the polymorphisms are found in the C4d segment of the C4 molecule chain. Several methods have been attempted to ascertain the C4 GCN, such as counting the number of fragments after restriction fragment length polymorphism (RFLP) analysis and densitometry of products obtained by Southern blotting and pulsed-field gel electrophoresis (PFGE). A multiplex ligation-dependent probe amplification (MLPA) assay in conjunction with isotype-specific ELISAs has been used to ascertain the level of C4A and C4B. Quantitative TaqMan real-time PCR (qPCR) tests were created using the breakpoint region of RP-C4-CYP21-TNX (RCCX) modular duplication, structural traits corresponding to long and short C4 genes, and nucleotide sequences specific for the C4A and C4B genes. Researchers described eight HLA haplotypes with single C4 genes in mono-modular RCCX that are linked to several autoimmune and infectious diseases, as well as 32 bi-modular, 4 tri-modular, and one quadri-modular RCCX, using cloned C4 genomic DNA (gDNA) covering six logs of DNA concentrations for calibration and a relative standard curve.

A fluorescent dye is added to the amplified DNA during the PCR process in a qPCR. The number of amplified copies determines how much light the dye emits. For tracking the kinetics of the amplification process, the TaqMan dye chemistry is unique and accurate(Navarro et al., 2015). The number of cycles needed to reach a threshold (CT), at which the fluorescence increases significantly and passes an arbitrarily defined value, is used to quantify the initial amount of DNA present in the reaction. Human genetic diversity is frequently seen in the form of single nucleotide polymorphisms (SNPs). Throughout the human genome, SNPs are biallelic and appear roughly every 1,000 base pairs (bp). SNPs are effective markers for mapping disease-causing genes. SNPs found in the major histocompatibility complex (MHC) have lately been linked to diseases like multiple sclerosis, diabetes, and rheumatoid arthritis that are known to be associated with HLA phenotypes and haplotypes. SNPs are easily genotyped using methods that distinguish between any two-way combination of adenine, guanine, cytosine, and thymine nucleotide bases due to their biallelic nature. Real-time quantitative assays are among the most reliable methods for SNP genotyping. They use polymerase chain reaction (PCR) to quantify amplified DNA or cDNA in a sensitive and specific manner. For the identification of genetic variation, real-time PCR techniques include a range of labels, including fluorogenic probes and DNA-intercalating agents. The technique can be applied to the genotyping of individual SNPs found in the human genome. TaqMan probes have a quencher dye or 6-carboxy-tetramethyl-rhodamine [TAMRA]) at the 3' end and a fluorescent reporter dye specific for alleles linked to the 5' end(Eun et al., 2000). A real-time PCR system or a thermal cycler is used for the amplification. Each individually labeled probe attaches preferentially to one of the two alleles of the target SNP with varying affinities during amplification. A fluorescent signal is produced when the Taq polymerase enzyme cleaves the attached probe during the amplification process. Sequence detection software specifically designed for real-time PCR equipment is used to automatically interpret fluorescent signals.

The trans-membrane ™ region typing has become more crucial for resolving ambiguities in major histocompatibility complex class I-related chain A (MICA) allele typing due to the large number of MICA alleles. Researchers have created a technique that uses the PCR products that are generated following generic MICA amplification of exons 2-5 to analyze MICA polymorphisms in exons 2-4 and the TM types in exon 5. This typing method eliminates short tandem repeats in the transmembrane region and employs computerized polymorphic site assignment. Without requiring any further steps, this approach can resolve any MICA allele and carry out MICA allele typing.

6.10 Data processing and statistics

The ability to produce immunogenetic data has much improved, but it is unclear whether the biostatistical ability to evaluate such large amounts of data has evolved similarly. Immunogenetics is unique in that it pertains to both fundamental and practical research domains. In certain situations, information about multiple people can appear on a single row of the master data file. In contrast, a single-subject observation is typically dispersed throughout multiple rows when the study design calls for repeated trials over time or under various conditions. This could be the case, for instance, when examining a trail consistency across several operators or approaches. A variable should be assigned to each column or field in the master data file. A variable is an observed or measured attribute that can have many values and that can be assigned a numerical value or a classification category. In the data set, it describes a single object. Every column should, if at all possible, have a number code, and any missing values also need to have a conventional code. Each variable should frequently have a brief but informative name, which is kept in the first row of each column (column header). Because they directly contain information, these variables are sometimes referred to as raw or primary variables; derived variables encode information that may be extracted from the raw variables and added to the master data file. Body mass index (BMI), for instance, can be computed using height and weight variables, but it could also be helpful to include a computed BMI in the master data file. Other variable fields that will contain variable data produced as part of the analyses may be included in the master data file. Redundancies between fields should generally be avoided in the design of the master data file. Identifying the type of variables included in the master data file is also crucial at this early stage of the analysis; the two most significant variable types are quantitative and qualitative, and the statistical approach chosen will rely on the kind of variable being examined.

6.11 Computational approaches

The majority of analytical techniques have not been specifically developed for immunogenetic data, although data analysis is a key component of contemporary genetic and genomic research approaches. The high level of polymorphism at the HLA and KIR loci requires analytical techniques and software tools that can process 20 or more alleles per locus for many loci(Nelson et al., 2015). The large linkage disequilibrium (LD) between immunogenetic loci necessitates the simultaneous calculation of association measures between up to 14 highly polymorphic loci such as in the KIR complex. Certain adjustments must occasionally be made in order to facilitate analysis because no single instrument can do all analyses and because the tools that are currently available are not ideal for immunogenetic data. Researchers and analysts should always observe that differences in terminology and data resolution might complicate analysis, even when an analytical application is suitable for the data. The analytical instruments do not yield fresh information or uncover facts; rather, they enable the application of sophisticated techniques, but the researcher should constantly be aware of and comprehend these techniques and their underlying presumptions. If an analytical finding is not given in the proper context, it should not be accepted. This reduces analyst error, makes it easier to explain what was done, and increases reproducibility for both the researcher and other researchers. Although software tools often run in one of three operating systems, Microsoft Windows, Apple, or Linux/Unix, or in a web browser, researchers do not suggest one above the others because many programs do not work in all three. To utilize all of the capabilities available, researchers should keep access to all three operating systems.

Due to their high CPU and memory requirements, many of these computations are computationally expensive. Modern computer systems should be capable of handling the tasks required to run the apps, but an analysis will proceed more quickly with the faster CPU and more RAM on a machine. To guarantee that any known software problems have been fixed, care should be taken to make sure that the most recent version of any application is utilized for analysis. There is no justification for depending on an obsolete version of any of the tools, they are all free. R, the language and environment for statistical computing, has been used to implement many of the studies. A fundamental component of scientific inquiry is the independent replication of published findings. Although the creation of experimental data is sometimes understood to be the main focus of replication, it is just as crucial that the analysis of that data be reproduced. Accurate and comprehensive reporting of the examined data is necessary to enable replication of analytical results. It is now known that the killer cell immunoglobulin-like receptors (KIR) loci and their HLA ligands play a part in solid organ and hematopoietic stem cell transplantation, pregnancy, autoimmune diseases, and infectious diseases (HIV and Hepatitis C). However, to prevent confusing results, special caution must be used when evaluating data for disease association studies due to the high levels of polymorphism associated with these loci. Although the majority of the analyses can be performed using commercial or customized computer software, none of the current programs, either separately or in combination, are capable of handling the complexity of the analyses required to identify primary and secondary disease genes in polymorphic immunogenetic regions. One of the main challenges in identifying certain causative genetic variants is the complex linkage disequilibrium (LD) patterns present in many immunogenetic studies. Some analysis algorithms only provide the evaluation of a small number of highly polymorphic loci, while others do not function with the high degree of polymorphism present in some locations, such as HLA. Our efforts to identify predisposing (PRE) genes for complicated diseases are made more difficult by the influence of environmental factors, age, and gender-specific effects, concealed disease heterogeneity, and gene-gene and gene-environment interactions. Therefore, researchers highly advise a multi-strategy approach that makes use of a range of complementary techniques.

6.12 Genetic studies

A vital population-based method for epidemiological research, such as genetic association studies, is case-control studies. These studies often include a control sample of unrelated, unaffected individuals selected from the same population, as well as samples of unrelated persons with the phenotype of interest. Immunogenetic studies generally recommend having at least 200 chromosomes in each of the case and control cohorts, though much larger sample sizes are preferred(Hollenbach et al., 2012). One benefit of case-control studies is that they do not require collecting data from family members, which can be expensive and logistically challenging. However, in immunogenetic data, where allele frequency distributions can differ significantly between human ethnic groups, case-control studies can be extremely sensitive to population stratification within the sample cohorts. Researchers risk misinterpreting genetic differences between patients and controls if samples are not gathered with meticulous attention to the homogeneity of ancestral background. In these situations, population stratification-related allele frequency discrepancies between cases and controls could be misconstrued for relation with a specific locus. The first step in any study involving immunogenetic data is population analyses, which include estimates of haplotype frequencies, tests for fit to expectations under Hardy-Weinberg Equilibrium (HWE), and calculations of gene (allele) frequencies. These analyses will give additional tools to evaluate any underlying population substructure and additional units of analysis on which association analyses will be conducted. Although there are many computer programs available to perform such calculations on genetic data, it is important to use tools specifically made for immunogenetic data or ones that can handle the high levels of polymorphism characteristic of these loci.

6.13 Graft and HLA

Graft survival rates have been increasing over the past few years, raising questions about whether organs should be distributed based on HLA compatibility or if kidneys from deceased donors should be transplanted locally with the shortest cold ischemia time possible, ignoring HLA matching. Some researchers discovered that transporting kidneys from deceased donors was linked to a higher probability of graft failure in the first year following transplantation in a survey of transplants where one kidney was transported and the other was placed locally. However, the improved physiological quality of donor organs recovered and transplanted locally may be the cause of this outcome rather than extended ischemia. Short cold ischemia does not negate the benefit of HLA matching, according to the results of the Collaborative Transplant Study(Süsal & Opelz, 2012). Better HLA matching in renal transplantation is linked to lower doses of immunosuppressive agents and a lower incidence of immunosuppressive side effects, such as non-Hodgkin lymphoma and hip fractures. Others have demonstrated that if a patient is relisted for a retransplant after losing kidney transplantation, greater HLA matching is linked to lower-grade sensitization. HLA matching may potentially help improve lung transplantation. Despite advancements in immunosuppression and a reduction in the duration of ischemic preservation, the impact of HLA matching on the survival rate of kidney transplants from deceased donors remains significant in a comparative analysis of over 130,000 deceased-donor kidney transplants carried out over two consecutive decades (1985-1994 and 1995-2004). The relative contribution of HLA mismatches to the fraction of graft failures stayed almost constant, even though the percentage increase in graft survival by HLA matching was lower in recent years.

6.14 Cross matches in transplantation

Overall, research studies revealed that no positive crossmatch or organ transplant type was associated with significant rates of hyperacute rejection, most likely as a result of advancements in immunosuppressive therapy. According to research studies on the first kidney transplant recipients, positive lymphocytotoxic T-cell crossmatches were linked to significantly lower graft survival. This suggests that specific selection and treatment strategies may have been successfully created and implemented in more recent years. Poor graft outcomes were linked to positive B-cell crossmatches. The percentage of positive crossmatches in kidney retransplants was roughly twice as high as the fraction of positive crossmatches in first transplants, highlighting the sensitizing effect of first graft rejection. Positive T-cell or B-cell crossmatches had a significantly greater impact on graft survival in retransplants than in initial grafts, and this effect was largely constant. Graft rejections in these patients might have been avoided with specific immunosuppressive therapy techniques. The percentage of positive T-cell crossmatches and positive B-cell crossmatches in heart transplant analysis was almost eight times and two times greater, respectively, than in kidney transplant studies. T-cell and B-cell crossmatches were linked to significantly worse heart transplant outcomes between 2000 and 2007 compared to the earlier 1990-1999 period(Norin et al., 2013). This could be because induction treatment, which uses powerful antibody agents (OKT3/ATG) to prevent graft rejection, has become less popular due to the elevated risk of post transplantation lymphoma that goes along with it. During the first time period (1990-1999), the fraction of positive crossmatches in liver transplantation was even higher than that in heart transplants, and it remained comparable in the more recent time period (2000-2007). Particularly during the most recent data period (2000-2007), positive T-cell crossmatches in liver transplantation were statistically linked to decreased graft survival.

There was no significant correlation seen between the outcome and positive B-cell crossmatches. Since early hyperacute graft rejection is uncommon and the consequences of a positive crossmatch are thus not immediately apparent, it is likely that most heart and liver transplants are still performed without a pre transplant crossmatch test. However, crossmatch-positive recipients have an increasing graft loss rate during the first three months of post-transplantation follow-up. The performance of pre-transplantation T-cell crossmatches in heart and liver transplantation is strongly supported by the CTS data. Prolonged organ preservation timeframes can typically be avoided because the crossmatch test can be conducted between the time of brain death declaration and the donor organ removal. A crossmatch-negative backup patient must be chosen for transplantation in the event of a positive crossmatch finding, which necessitates logistical planning. Additional strategies for lowering the frequency of positive crossmatch outcomes in heart and liver transplants include pre-transplantation characterization of the recipient alloantibodies and subsequent virtual crossmatching. Compared to the conventional cell-based techniques, solid-phase immunoassays offer higher sensitivity, specificity, time, and reagent efficiency for the detection and characterization of HLA-specific antibodies. Test kits that are sold commercially are used for testing. Multianalyte beads and enzyme-linked immunosorbent assays are the two main categories of tests. Although these assays are a significant advance over cell-based assays, interfering compounds in the blood that cause high background reactivity can confuse them. Because of their high sensitivity, the tests are also more susceptible to operator error and environmental influences.

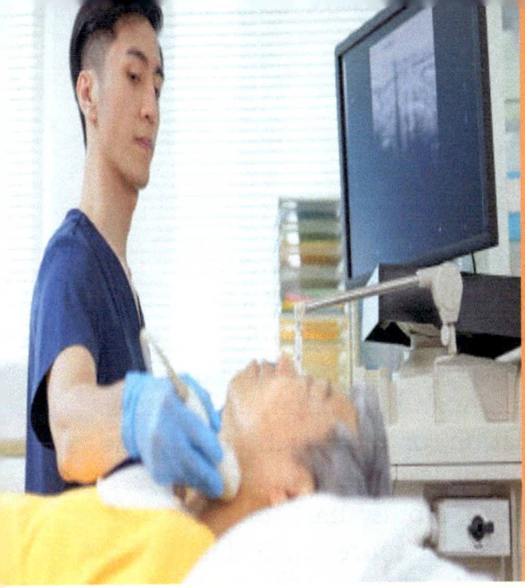

Chapter 7

ENDOCRINOLOGY AND AUTOIMMUNITY

Contents

7.1 Introduction

Many diseases that impact one or more endocrine glands are included in the category of autoimmune endocrinopathies. Their pathophysiology involves environmental influences as well as a significant genetic tendency that drives their growth. These environmental agents include radiation, chemicals, infections, and drugs. Since exposure to these environmental factors frequently occurs before the start of disease, it is challenging to establish a clear link between them and autoimmune diseases. Changes in autologous antigens, modifications to immune modulation, or modifications to gene expression are some of the pathways that might trigger autoimmunity. Environmental influences, which can be controlled by the type, amount, and length of exposure, modify immune responses based on the host's genetic vulnerability. Many diseases involving one or more endocrine glands are included in the category of autoimmune endocrinopathies. They develop due to a hereditary predisposition, just as the majority of autoimmune disorders. Astute clinician observations of clustering of thyroid and other endocrine organ diseases in specific families provided the first indication that these diseases have a genetic component.

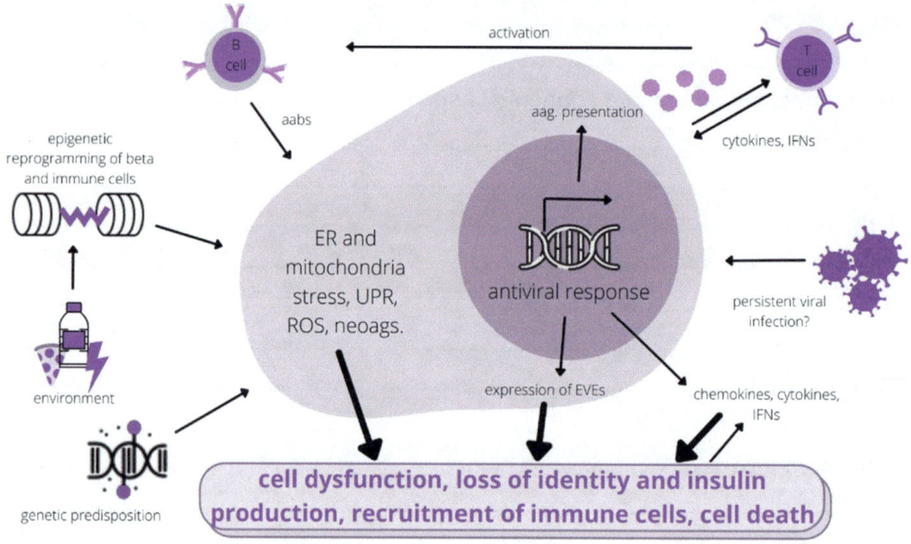

Figure 7.1 Type 1 diabetes mellitus

Source: Zajec, A., Trebušak Podkrajšek, K., Tesovnik, T., Šket, R., Čugalj Kern, B., Jenko Bizjan, B., Šmigoc Schweiger, D., Battelino, T., & Kovač, J. (2022). Pathogenesis of Type 1 Diabetes: Established Facts and New Insights. Genes, 13(4), 706. https://doi.org/10.3390/genes13040706,*Creative Commons License.*

Type 1 diabetes mellitus (T1DM) (Figure 7.1) was more common among the siblings and children of T1DM patients than in the general population(Murillo et al., 2017). Large-scale investigations demonstrate that relatives of patients with autoimmune endocrine disease frequently have antibodies to the same or different endocrine organs. Research studies have linked the major histocompatibility complex (MHC) to autoimmune endocrinopathy development as a key genetic risk factor. Recent research has identified several immunoregulatory genes, including the lymphoid tyrosine phosphatase locus (LYP/PTPN22) and the cytotoxic T-lymphocyte-associated antigen (CTLA)-4, that increase vulnerability to specific autoimmune diseases of the endocrine organs. The genetic characteristics that increase the target organ susceptibility have been identified. The recognition of immunodominant, pathogenic epitopes, traits that alter the immune response, and inherited traits that predispose to harmful inflammation in the target organ are the main gene categories that appear to play a role in determining inherited susceptibility to autoimmune disease. Several years ago, researchers hypothesized that the best model for explaining the genetic predisposition to autoimmune disease is the accumulation of several unrelated genetic traits that contribute to susceptibility to autoimmune-mediated tissue injury by various pathways.

7.2 Etiologies

Artificial breeding of disease-susceptibility genes has resulted in models of spontaneous autoimmune endocrinopathy in experimental animals. These comprise the obese strain (OS) chicken and NOD.H2h4 mouse model of Hashimoto's thyroiditis or the non-obese diabetic (NOD) mice model of type 1 diabetes. In contrast, it seems that less than half of the sensitivity to autoimmune disease in humans can be attributed to genetic predisposition overall. The etiology of autoimmune endocrinopathies involves both genetic and environmental variables, as seen by the 5-50% concurrence rates for T1DM and autoimmune thyroid disease in genetically identical twins. The immune system lymphocyte receptors experience significant post-germline recombination throughout the diversification process. Even genetically identical mice or monozygotic twins can have very different immune recognition. Other endocrine and neurological system regulatory actions impact the immune response. As a result, women are far more likely than men to suffer from a variety of autoimmune diseases, particularly those affected by thyroid. These diseases might be absent during pregnancy, but they might come back and get worse after giving birth. The immune response is also influenced by nervous signals, such as stress. Therefore, immunologic alterations may contribute to the comparatively low concordance rates in monozygotic twins rather than only environmental influences. However, epidemiologic research supports the idea that environmental factors do contribute significantly to the development of autoimmune diseases. For instance, in both the northern and southern hemispheres, the onset of clinical type 1 diabetes is lower in the summer than in the winter. With no discernible link to genetic variations, the incidence or prevalence of T1DM is generally higher in southern Australian states than in northern states and higher in northern European countries than in southern states. Over the past three to five decades, the frequency of type 1 diabetes has increased significantly in several countries, coinciding with a decline in the age at which the condition first manifests and an expansion of the risk profile associated with the human leukocyte antigen (HLA). These findings imply that a growing percentage of genetically susceptible people are influenced by their surroundings.

7.3 Environmental factors and congenital aspects

The environmental variables have a role in the genesis of autoimmune diseases, particularly those affecting the endocrine system. There are theories that infection contributes directly or indirectly to the etiology of autoimmune diseases because these conditions often develop after infection. The adjuvant effect of infection occurs when infections create the inflammatory environment that makes self-antigens more potent. Proinflammatory cytokine production and costimulatory molecule upregulation can both be caused by infectious agents. The autoreactive T cells can initiate an autoimmune reaction. A change in the Th1/Th2 equilibrium brought on by infections can occasionally encourage the development of pathogenic rather than benign autoimmunity(Hart et al., 2015). Infection might change self-antigens or cause them to manifest in a way that increases their immunogenic potential. Molecular mimicry occurs when the epitopes on specific pathogens resemble the epitopes on self-antigens, triggering an autoimmune reaction. A correlation between infectious pathogens and autoimmune disorders is hard to establish. Autoimmune diseases can develop considerably later than infections. An autoimmune reaction frequently takes months or years to manifest clinically once it has begun. As a result, an infant infection might not manifest as an autoimmune disease until adolescence or early adulthood. Only those who are genetically more vulnerable, as identified by non-HLA and HLA genes, may be affected by an infectious agent and develop autoimmune disease.

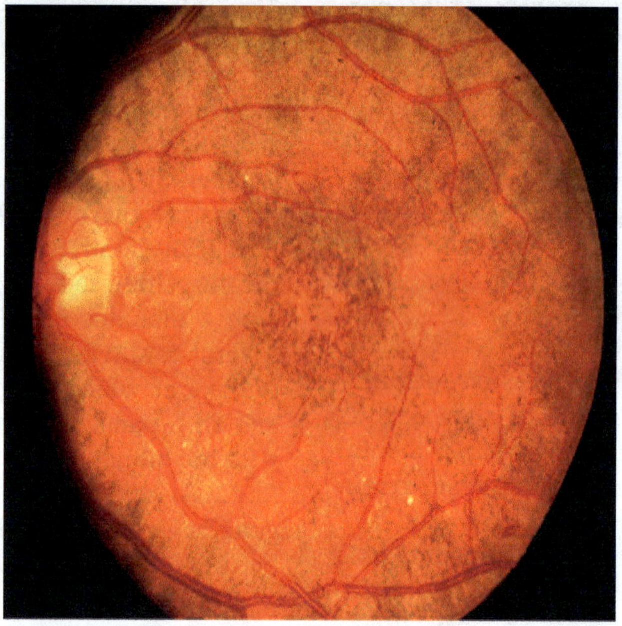

Figure 7.2 Congenital rubella syndrome

Source: https://upload.wikimedia.org/wikipedia/commons/c/c0/Congenital_Rubella_Syndrome%2C_Salt_and_Pepper_Retinopathy.jpg,*Creative Commons License.*

In people with extremely predisposed genetic backgrounds, an infection may not increase the likelihood of developing an autoimmune disease. In patients with a reduced genetic predisposition, the cumulative effect of infection may raise the risk of developing autoimmune disease. Some researchers have shown that only the genetically low-risk population lacking the high-risk HLA had a seasonal increase in T1DM. Many infections have a high probability of causing benign autoimmune reactions, such as autoantibodies. What causes certain patients to develop a full-blown autoimmune disease is yet unknown. Some autoimmune diseases have become more common in recent decades. Since no significant genetic changes take place in the population in short, environmental factors are most likely responsible for this growth. The first potential environmental factor is viral infections. Many research studies examined various viruses in an attempt to explain the rise in the incidence of T1DM. An enterovirus infection is one of the primary causes of type 1 diabetes. Nonetheless, it is known that Finland saw a decline in enterovirus infection rates during the 1980s and 1990s. Whereas the prevalence of type 1 diabetes rose in Finland, it stayed constant in the genetically comparable populations of Estonia and Russian Karelia(Knip et al., 2017). Many investigations reveal the existence of autoantibodies after an infectious disease has started, which is not proof of the cause. The question of whether a single virus infection might raise the incidence of an autoimmune disease can only be addressed by longitudinal, HLA-matched research. Different viruses may cause the same autoimmune disease in people if viral infections, as demonstrated in mice, function as adjuvants in the development of autoimmune diseases.

We know that congenital rubella syndrome (CRS) (Figure 7.2) is associated with an increased risk of T1DM and thyroid disorders. Patients may experience growth hormone deficiency and Addison's disease, among other endocrine disorders. The pancreas and other fetal tissues can be used to isolate the rubella virus. T1DM can develop in up to 20% of fetuses infected with rubella. Initially, it was believed that rubella started the autoimmune process that destroyed islet cells. It has been documented that T lymphocytes from CRS patients recognize glutamic acid decarboxylase (GAD) determinants and have a relationship with the HLA haplotype DR3. Diabetes-associated autoantibodies were detected in 20% of CRS patients. In an investigation of 37 CRS patients from Finland and Poland, no diabetes-associated autoantibodies, including GAD, insulin autoantibodies (IAA), islet cell antibodies (ICA), or IA-2a, were found. Since the rubella vaccine was introduced in the US in 1969, the incidence of rubella infection in fetuses has dropped by 99 percent. This reduction in fetal rubella exposure did not stop the rise in the prevalence of diabetes in the general population, indicating that rubella is not the primary cause of most diabetes cases. It appears that rather than being caused by an autoimmune mechanism, diabetes in CRS may primarily arise following the death of the pancreatic beta cells.

7.4 Mumps and diabetes

Mumps and diabetes have long been linked in several publications. Some reports raised the possibility of a link between a higher incidence of T1DM two to four years after contracting mumps. Since then, autoimmune diabetes and mumps have been connected in many cases. According to one study, seven children who contracted active mumps after immunization and 127 children who got the disease naturally developed antibodies against islet cells but showed no signs of disease(Rubin & Kennedy, 2020). Human beta cells in vitro infected with the mumps virus produce more proinflammatory cytokines and expression of HLA class I got upregulated. There was a halt in the rising incidence of type 1 diabetes in Finland with the introduction of the mumps, measles, and rubella (MMR) immunization in 1982, but this halt was only temporary. T1DM incidence did not generally decline with the introduction of the mumps vaccine. It is still unknown whether mumps virus infection and type 1 diabetes are related. Some members of the enterovirus family are pancreotropic and can damage islet cells. Neutralizing antibodies revealed an Echovirus 6 infection in the mother at 14 weeks of pregnancy, which was linked to a case of neonatal diabetes. The baby had antibodies to GAD and insulin, while the mother did not. A patient who died soon after developing acute type 1 diabetes had Coxsackievirus B (CB) 4 identified from their pancreas. The autopsy revealed beta-cell necrosis and lymphocytic infiltration of the pancreatic islet cells. The titer increased from less than 4 on day 2 to 32 on the day of death, according to serologic data. Within a few days, mice infected with the virus linked to this patient developed serious diabetes. The beta cell injury was linked to CB4-specific antigens in the islets. RNA hybridization in the beta cells of babies who died from fulminant disease indicates that the Coxsackievirus can replicate in human beta cells.

As early as 24 hours after infection, a reduction in insulin output was observed, indicating that the virus cocultivation with pancreatic beta cells hindered islet metabolism. These findings demonstrate the high potential for enteroviruses to damage the pancreas and result in diabetes in humans or animals. However, they do not demonstrate that an autoimmune reaction is the source of the disease. Many epidemiologic studies show that patients are more likely than healthy controls to have antienterovirus immunoglobulin (Ig)M antibodies at the beginning of diabetes. Serum from T1DM patients has also been found to contain enteroviral RNA. A study of diabetics in Sweden using a molecular method using PCR of peripheral blood mononuclear cells revealed that 50% of the individuals had evidence of CB4, CB5, and CB6 in contrast to 26% of normal siblings who had no infection in age and sex-matched normal controls. Evidence of virus-specific IgM responses to CB4 and CB5 during the juvenile onset of type 1 diabetes is presented by other studies involving patients from England, Austria, and Australia. Some researchers evaluated T cell proliferation to viral proteins and demonstrated a correlation between MHC II, CB infection, and T1DM. According to these investigations, enterovirus infections can occur before diabetes develops. The possibility that prediabetic patients with persistent but clinically silent diabetes are more likely to contract CB3 infection or that their genetic composition predisposes them to both diabetes and enterovirus infection separately is not disregarded, though. HLA-DR3 or HLA-DR4 positivity is, in fact, more common in diabetic patients with anti-CB3 IgM antibodies than in controls. In the six months before the onset of ICA, enterovirus infections were identified in 51% of cases and 28% of controls in a longitudinal diabetes prevention study conducted in Finland(Honkanen et al., 2017). Other longitudinal investigations conducted in Australia and the United States failed to find any link between enteroviral infection and the development of islet cell autoimmunity or diabetes symptoms. The findings could be attributed to changes in the viruses, the geographic spread of the disease, the ages of the populations under study, or the genetic backgrounds of the populations.

7.5 Viral infections

Animal models show that the CB3 infection may have the ability to accelerate an autoimmune process that is already underway. In the NOD model of autoimmune diabetes, it has been shown that whereas pre-insulitis CB infection prevents the development of diabetes, infection eight weeks after insulitis onset speeds up the start of disease. Although the destruction of the thyroid gland can result in hypothyroidism, viruses are thought to be the cause of subacute thyroiditis, which typically lasts a few weeks and declines on its own. Clinical signs of subacute thyroiditis include follicular epithelium breakdown, hoarseness and thyrotoxicosis symptoms, dysphagia, and painful thyroid gland enlargement. One possibility in subacute thyroiditis is mumps infection. The measles virus, Epstein-Barr virus (EBV), influenza, adenovirus, and enteroviruses are viruses that may be responsible for subacute thyroiditis. Half of the patients with subacute thyroiditis had altered antibody titers against some viruses, including the mumps and influenza. Recent research did not corroborate these findings. Some patients with subacute thyroiditis showed no changes in antiviral antibody titers against chicken pox, mumps, measles, parvovirus B19, cytomegalovirus (CMV), rubella, or type I herpes. No EBV or CMV DNA was found in these patients (thyroid). Therefore, it appears that subacute thyroiditis can be caused by a variety of viruses. It is unclear, therefore, how autoimmunity contributes to the pathophysiology of the disease.

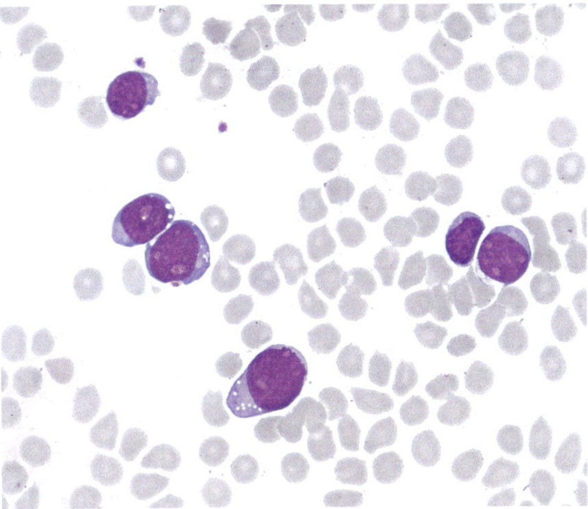

Figure 7.3 T-cell leukemia

Source: https://upload.wikimedia.org/wikipedia/commons/c/c3/T-ALL_cells.jpg,*Creative Commons License.*

The autoimmune component might be a general reaction to inflammation and thyroid antigen release. Most cases of subacute thyroiditis go away on their own without developing into the more common autoimmune form. Many viral infections can occasionally be linked to autoimmune thyroid disease, including Hashimoto's and Graves' diseases. There is currently conflicting evidence linking a chronic hepatitis C virus or HCV infection of the liver to a number of autoimmune disorders, including autoimmune thyroiditis. Prior to interferon therapy, a number of investigations discovered that HCV patients had hypothyroidism and elevated antithyroid antibodies. It is unclear if HCV can interact with other environmental factors or if, as some research would indicate, the risk of thyroiditis is elevated primarily in a subset of the HCV population, such as older females.

7.6 Retroviruses and other pathogens

Retroviruses are responsible for the production of autoimmune thyroid disease. T-cell leukemia (Figure 7.3) is thought to be caused by the human retrovirus known as human T-cell leukemia virus type I (HTLV-I), which is very prevalent in southern Japan, Latin America, tropical Africa, Melanesia, and the Caribbean. It was demonstrated that a higher than anticipated number of Hashimoto's patients had HTLV-1 positive. Anti-thyroid antibodies are also more common in HTLV-1 carriers than in the normal population. The HTLV-I envelope protein and DNA were found in the thyroid follicular epithelial cells of a patient with Graves' disease and Hashimoto's thyroiditis. For many years, autoimmune thyroid disease has been thought to be caused or triggered by a chronic infection with *Yersinia enterocolitica*. Patients with thyroid disease had a high prevalence of Yersinia antibodies. Of the patients, 83% had Hashimoto's thyroiditis and 66% had Graves' disease. In contrast to 8% of controls, all individuals tested positive for Yersinia antibodies. Cross-reaction between thyroid antibodies and Yersinia antigens caused this. Research of 30 twins revealed a higher incidence of antibodies to Yersinia serotype 3 in thyroid patients, further supporting the link between Graves' disease and Yersinia infection(Brix et al., 2008). Leukocyte migration inhibition tests have shown that leukocytes from patients with Graves' disease may also identify Yersinia antigens. The discovery of a thyroid-stimulating hormone (TSH) binding site on *Yersinia enterocolitica* raises the possibility of a mechanism connecting the two diseases. Human thyrotropin receptors have been demonstrated to interact with purified antibodies to *Y. enterocolitica* envelope proteins. Following Yersinia vaccination, mice developed antibodies against the thyrotropin receptor. One possible instance of molecular mimicry is the interaction between *Y. enterocolitica* epitopes and the human thyrotropin receptor. It is still unknown if Yersinia infection causes autoimmune thyroid disease in susceptible people or if it only results in temporary anti-TSH-R antibodies. The correlation between infection with Helicobacter pylori and autoimmune thyroid disease has been also hypothesized. Compared to the control group, thyroid patients had a high prevalence of positive *H. pylori* antibodies. Individual HLA haplotypes and Helicobacter serology did not correlate.

The evidence is insufficient to determine whether the increased *H. pylori* infection is due to the same genetic susceptibility factors or whether *H. pylori* play any causal role in the pathophysiology of thyroiditis. Autoantibodies generated as the result of parasite infections are generally polyreactive, binding to several self-antigens as well as external antigens. Although several instances of the relationship of parasite infections with other autoimmune disorders are cited in the literature, only a few examples have been described for the autoimmune endocrinopathies. According to some investigations, there was no association between abnormal blood thyroxine (T4) or serum triiodothyronine (T3) levels and 17 men afflicted with schistosomiasis. By changing the Th1/Th2 responses, infectious pathogens can also affect the pathophysiology of the disease. The hygiene hypothesis explains how environmental influences can further change these responses. In a mouse model of Graves' disease, another study reports immunological polarization brought on by schistosomiasis infection. Since galactosylceramide is known to bias immunity toward Th2 responses, it was employed as a synthetic glycolipid. The helminth infection is a Th1-dominant disease rather than a Th2. Neither infection nor α-galactosylceramide was able to decrease disease after the thyrotropin receptor response was fully established, indicating that the timing of antigen priming is critical in connection to infection. It becomes challenging to block pathogenic responses after antigen priming has begun. Mixed Th1/Th2 responses are seen in all autoimmune endocrinopathies.

Therefore, it is challenging to link these reactions to a particular autoimmune condition. IgG antibodies against measles, mumps, or both were observed to have an inhibitory effect on the prevalence of thyroperoxidase antibodies in comparison to seronegative controls. For rubella antibodies, no such link was discovered. The prevalence of islet cell antibodies in the group that tested positive for measles, mumps, or rubella did not alter. There were no thyroid conditions among the children. The future development of autoimmune thyroiditis in children with thyroid antibodies is uncertain, as is the potential protective effect of vaccinations or infections against measles or mumps against thyroid disease.

7.7 Thyroid dysfunction

While thyroid dysfunction linked to thalidomide, betaroxine, stavudine, lithium carbonate, aminoglutethimide, and amiodarone is well known, glucose intolerance has been linked in some patients to recent or concurrent exposures to drugs such as beta-blockers, thiazide diuretics, and antipsychotics. Fewer drugs have been clinically linked to autoimmune thyroiditis, T1DM, and autoimmune endocrinopathies.

7.8 STZ-based studies

The tacrolimus, Vacor, cyclosporine, and streptozotocin (STZ) have all been linked to the rapid development of diabetes with features similar to type 1 diabetes. Hypothyroidism with autoimmune characteristics has been linked to amiodarone, interleukin (IL), and interferon (IFN)-α(Cyna et al., 2024). The emergence of autoimmune endocrinopathies in these patients has led physicians to question whether the drug is the main trigger or if the patient has an autoimmune endocrinopathy risk that was previously unknown. Several drugs linked with autoimmune endocrinopathies in patients have also been related to the production of diabetes and autoimmune thyroiditis in animal models of these disorders. These drug-induced animal models of autoimmune thyroiditis or diabetes have shed light on potential processes linked to the onset of autoimmune endocrinopathies in humans. Though hyperglycemia and glucose intolerance have been reported in several patients, STZ, a glucosamine nitrosourea compound, has been used for many years as a broad-spectrum antibiotic and more recently as a chemotherapeutic agent for neuroendocrine tumors. Subsequent research showed that two STZ regimens, one administered approximately two to three days after a single high-dose (90 mg/kg) intraperitoneal injection, or five to six days after five daily low-dose (40 mg/kg) intraperitoneal injections of this compound, can cause insulin-dependent diabetes in mice(Yuan et al., 2016). Both regimens have been employed in STZ-diabetes model experiments. Multiple doses of STZ, however, might be less harmful to the mice receiving this experimental regimen. Researchers concur that the animal model of insulin-dependent diabetes offers a unique chance to examine potential mechanisms underlying T1DM in humans. It also serves as a means of examining how this autoimmune endocrinopathy contributes to the development of diabetic nephropathy, complications during pregnancy, and rejection or tolerance of pancreatic islet cells.

Several strains of mice have been discovered to be susceptible to STZ-induced insulin-dependent diabetes. These mice include diabetes-susceptible NOD mice before the beginning of spontaneous insulinitis male CD-1 mice, and male mice administered low doses of STZ (MSZ). Testosterone was linked to a hyperglycemic reaction in susceptible male mice compared to female mice. Therefore, the effect of gender and genetics in the development of diabetes might also be studied using the STZ model of diabetes in mice. Although most studies concur that direct damage to pancreatic beta cells is the pathway responsible for diabetes following STZ administration, no one mechanism has been able to fully explain the development of insulin-dependent diabetes in mice after STZ administration. Although the exact mechanism causing the death of pancreatic beta cells is unknown, research has indicated that several immunological and non-immune systems may be crucial to this process. The widely accepted non-immune mechanism is based on the discovery that STZ is taken up by the glucose transporter Glut-2 in pancreatic beta cells. Research work showed that Glu-2 absorption of STZ caused either direct DNA damage by alkylation or indirect DNA damage once nitric oxide (NO) was generated. Pancreatic beta cell damage is caused by STZ-induced elevations in CD8+ T cell and macrophage counts, as well as cytokine damage from IFN-producing T-helper and cytotoxic T cells, due to the dominant immunological mechanism of STZ-induced insulin-dependent diabetes. Studies that further characterize these infiltrating T cells reveal that the T cells that infiltrate the islets of mice with STZ-induced diabetes are comparatively oligoclonal and express the Vβ.2 T-cell receptor. They also demonstrate that T cells from mice treated with STZ can transfer diabetes to naïve mice. Research studies examining the function of T-cell signaling in STZ-induced experimental diabetes have discovered that CD28 costimulation and T-cell self-recognition in inflammatory pancreatic islets are necessary for this condition. By producing oxygen-free radicals, these same macrophages can damage beta cells in the pancreas. Increased expression of inducible NO synthase, which leads to the synthesis of NO and peroxynitrite, is another mechanism that could be responsible for the generation of oxygen-free radicals. According to these investigations, the pathophysiology of STZ-induced experimental diabetes stops with the generation of oxygen-free radicals.

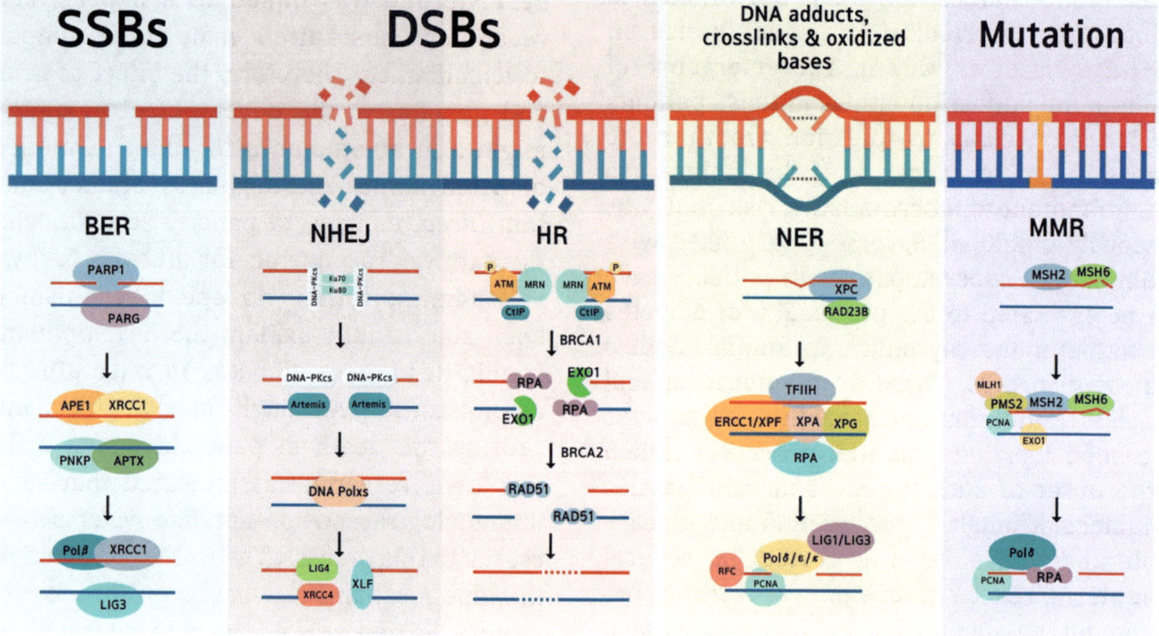

Figure 7.4 DNA damage

Source: Moon, J., Kitty, I., Renata, K., Qin, S., Zhao, F., & Kim, W. (2023). DNA Damage and Its Role in Cancer Therapeutics. International Journal of Molecular Sciences, 24(5), 4741. https://doi.org/10.3390/ijms24054741,*Creative Commons License.*

7.9 DNA damage

The significance of a non-immune mechanism involving direct DNA damage (Figure 7.4) and subsequent repair has been thoroughly studied in the past several years. These investigations may have been prompted by the finding that NO can functionally inhibit beta cells, leading to increased DNA damage, decreased insulin secretion, cell death, and decreased ATP levels. Research indicates that poly (ADP-ribose) synthase, also known as poly (ADP-ribose) polymerase, plays a crucial role in DNA repair in the mechanism of STZ-induced damage. These investigations also raise the possibility that they will identify potential treatment targets for individuals with type 1 diabetes in the future. An effective immunosuppressive drug, cyclosporin A (CSA) is a fungal metabolite that is mainly administered to patients following organ donation. CSA suppresses the immune system by first attaching to intracellular cyclophilin and then to calcium-dependent calcineurin. This binding to calcineurin stops the IL-2 gene from being activated, which stops T-cell clones from growing by interfering with the proliferating T-cell ability to produce IL-2(Duré & Macian, 2009). CSA has been linked to organ-specific autoimmune disease in experimental animals, glucose intolerance, type 1 diabetes, and subacute thyroiditis in humans after transplantation, despite its involvement in immunosuppression. Exact mechanisms responsible for CSA-associated autoimmune endocrinopathies in patients have not been thoroughly defined. Mechanisms for CSA-induced, organ-specific autoimmunity in mice have been studied.

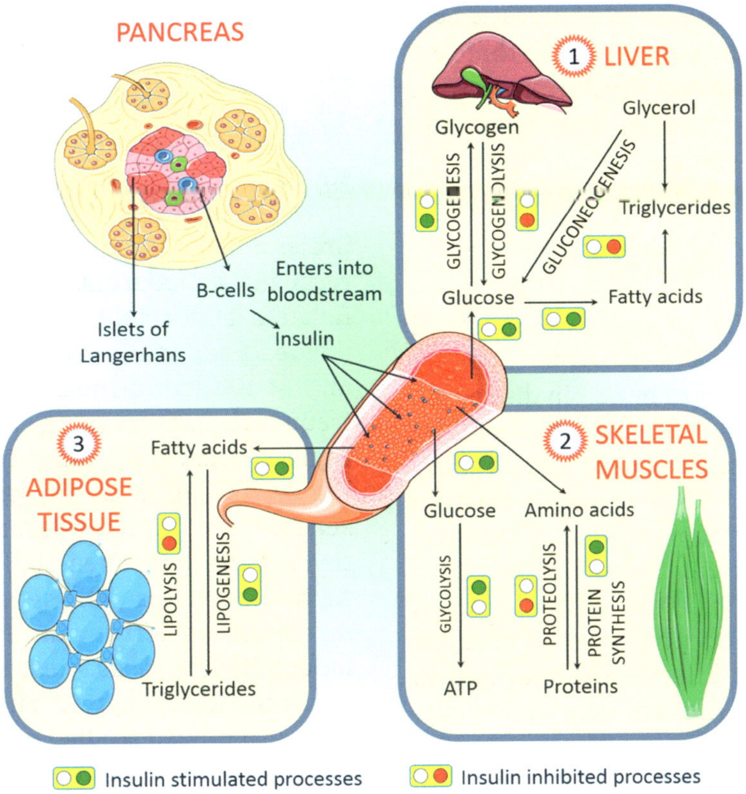

Figure 7.5 Insulin DNA

Source: Rahman, M. S., Hossain, K. S., Das, S., Kundu, S., Adegoke, E. O., Rahman, M. A., Hannan, M. A., Uddin, M. J., & Pang, M. -G. (2021). Role of Insulin in Health and Disease: An Update. International Journal of Molecular Sciences, 22(12), 6403. https://doi.org/10.3390/ijms22126403,*Creative Commons License.*

Researchers have discovered that giving CSA to newborn BALB/c mice daily causes gastritis, adrenalitis, insulinitis, and thyroiditis, along with the serum autoantibodies linked to these conditions, one or two weeks after stopping CSA treatments. A selective lack of regulatory T cells led to the development of organ-specific autoimmunity. Subsequent research revealed that CSA can cause thymic involution, delay the deletion of low-affinity thymic clones, or stop T-cell clonal anergy from developing, among other potential pathways that could possibly be responsible for CSA-induced autoimmunity. These researchers also pointed out that stopping CSA can cause a graft-versus-host reaction, which can exacerbate or cause autoimmune conditions like autoimmune thyroiditis.

According to earlier studies, T cells and T-cell function are the focus of the mechanism causing CSA-induced autoimmune endocrinopathy. The effects of CSA on pancreatic beta cell activity have been the main focus of other researchers looking into the processes behind the autoimmune endocrinopathy, T1DM, that is caused by CSA. Using in vitro cell cultures of rat pancreatic beta cells, these researchers demonstrated that CSA decreased glucose-induced insulin production and proposed some potential reasons for the decreased insulin secretion.

7.10 Other drugs

Insulin DNA (Figure 7.5) or mRNA was inhibited by CSA in the first method, while pancreatic beta cells were directly damaged by CSA in the second method. By interfering with the mitochondrial permeability transition pore, researchers demonstrated that CSA reduced insulin secretion. They also proposed that calcineurin was responsible for the immunosuppressive effects of CSA, while the mitochondrial permeability transition pore was responsible for the diabetogenic effects. The mechanism of CSA-induced autoimmune thyroiditis has not been as extensively investigated as that of T1DM, because a direct relationship with autoimmune thyroiditis in patients may be less evident. The mechanisms responsible for tacrolimus-induced T1DM in patients have not been fully understood. Previous investigations have indicated direct toxicity to pancreatic beta cells, decreased insulin sensitivity or decreased insulin release, or synthesis by pancreatic beta cells as probable pathways to explain this result. It will be beneficial to thoroughly examine these pathways in experimental animal models. Tacrolimus-induced autoimmune thyroiditis in humans has not yet been documented. A benzofuranic derivative called amiodarone is used to treat tachyarrhythmias in patients, including congestive heart failure and paroxysmal supraventricular tachycardia. Its comparatively long half-life of about 40 days and wide distribution to multiple tissues, such as the liver, heart, and thyroid, are just some of its distinctive pharmacological characteristics. Aside from these characteristics, it has a high iodine content that ranges from 27% to 37%, which causes patients receiving amiodarone treatment for extended periods to be exposed to more iodine(Eskes & Wiersinga, 2009). The amiodarone treatment has been linked to thyroid dysfunction; nevertheless, it is still debatable if amiodarone might result in thyroid autoimmunity. The majority of medical professionals concur that 14-18% of patients receiving amiodarone will experience thyroid function abnormalities, which can be broadly divided into some categories. Thyrotoxicosis, an amiodarone-induced abnormality, is frequently observed in male patients with thyroid disorders and is brought on by the deiodination of thyroxine, which raises serum-free T4. Amiodarone directly affects thyroid cells through iodine-induced excess thyroid hormone (TH) synthesis, which is the mechanism underlying this form of amiodarone-induced thyrotoxicosis, also known as AIT-1. The involvement of thyroid autoimmunity in this disease has been studied because these patients have underlying thyroid abnormalities. Based on these investigations, scientists concluded that in individuals without underlying thyroid conditions, humoral thyroid autoimmunity had no bearing on AIT-1. In patients who have no known thyroid problems, the second type of AIT, known as AIT-2, causes damaging thyroiditis due to the release of preformed hormones. Thyroid autoimmunity is not a problem in the AIT-2 condition.

The amiodarone-induced thyroid damage induces hypothyroidism and occurs more frequently in women with pre-existing thyroid damage, especially autoimmune thyroiditis. According to research on the etiology of amiodarone-induced hypothyroidism (AIH), amiodarone damage occurs in regions that have previously been damaged by autoimmune thyroiditis, making the patient more susceptible to iodine suppression of TH and unable to avoid the Wolff-Chaikoff effect. The link between AIH and autoimmune is based on an existing autoimmunity diagnosis rather than the emergence of new autoimmunity. These processes make it evident that amiodarone can cause thyroid damage; nevertheless, an already damaged thyroid gland may be necessary for the development of thyroid autoimmunity. After beginning amiodarone therapy, approximately 55% of patients produced these autoantibodies; however, subsequent researchers were unable to replicate these observations or experiments in other patient groups. Both patients and rodents can develop diabetes as a result of the rodenticide Vacor. Before 1993, people experienced symptoms resembling those of type 1 diabetes after unintentional or deliberate exposure to Vacor. In addition to potential direct suppression of NADH, the pathophysiology of diabetes in individuals or animals is believed to result from direct damage to pancreatic beta cells via mechanisms similar to those observed after STZ treatment. However, there is still a problem with autoimmunity after Vacor exposure.

7.11 Cells and cytokines

Two classes of IFNs can be distinguished: Type 1, which comprises IFN-α and IFN-β, and Type 2, which comprises IFN-γ(Kotenko, 2011). Researchers have found multiple type 1 alpha IFNs but just one type 1 beta IFN, which may indicate that IFN-γ may react to more environmental stimuli. Research has shown that IFN-γ can be induced in difficult experimental setups containing bacteria or lipopolysaccharide polyanions in addition to double-stranded DNA and IL-2, hypoxia, RNA, or vasoactive intestinal polypeptide. Researchers agree that viruses are the most powerful IFN-α inducers. Because of its many therapeutic benefits, IFN-α is also used to treat lymphomas, carcinoid tumors, leukemias, and breast cancer. Its antiviral qualities have thus been employed to treat chronic hepatitis B and C infections. Specific cell types including natural killer cells and monocytes as well as a variety of cytokines like IL-1, IL-2, IL-10, IL-4, IL-6, IL-8, and IL-15 can be used in various ways to generate these immune responses. Therefore, some patients receiving recombinant versions of these drugs or individuals with high IFN-α may be susceptible to developing autoimmune diseases due to IFN-α capacity to respond to a range of stimuli and elicit different effects on the immune system. Systemic lupus erythematosus (SLE), type 1 diabetes, and thyroiditis are among the autoimmune disorders that have been linked in the past to the injection of recombinant IFN-α and the induction of natural IFN-α. SLE is the most documented of the autoimmune diseases. It was evident from cross-sectional human research that SLE patients had higher serum IFN-α levels. It is interesting to note that these investigations did not show that these patient IFN-α levels increased with time. Pancreatic biopsies from patients recently diagnosed with type 1 diabetes likewise showed elevated levels of natural IFN-α, however like SLE, the increase was not consistent. Unlike these conditions, autoimmune thyroiditis has not been linked to increased expression of natural IFN-α, although it has been linked to psoriasis and celiac disease. IFN-α associated autoimmune thyroiditis is 6% more common than SLE and T1DM(Devendra & Eisenbarth, 2004). The risk factors for autoimmune thyroid diseases are similar to those linked to the development of type 1 diabetes after IFN-α; these include female sex, hepatitis C or cancer, thyroid autoantibodies that already existed, prolonged IFN-α therapy, or therapy in conjunction with IL-2. The thyroiditis may not resolve in some patients with hyperthyroidism who require therapy for more than five years. Research examining this phenomenon in hepatitis C patients suggested that, after recombinant IFN-α, autoimmune thyroiditis in the majority of patients spontaneously resolves. Identification of potential mechanisms underlying IFN-associated autoimmunity in patients has been aided by animal models of IFN-induced autoimmunity. It is evident from the animal model of IFN-α induced type 1 diabetes that pancreatic islets cells produce more IFN-α before diabetes develops in mice treated with STZ. Giving these mice anti-IFN-antibodies may stop them from developing diabetes. In mice treated with STZ, immunization with polyinosine/cytosine, an IFN-α inducing agent, accelerated the development of type 1 diabetes.

Experimental cancer vaccines have been administered with low-dose IL-2 as a systemic adjuvant. Antigen-specific T cell proliferation is another function of IL-2. However, autoimmune conditions like thyroiditis, T1DM, and vitiligo have been linked to IL-2 injection. According to some studies assessing the emergence of autoimmune diseases in patients receiving low-dose IL-2 and anti-tumor vaccines, autoimmune thyroiditis was the most prevalent autoimmune disease linked to this treatment.

Autoantibodies were not regularly assessed in the thyroiditis case both prior to and during the course of treatment. Anti-microsomal and anti-thyroglobulin (Tg) antibodies were found in some cases. Autoantibodies were not found in patients who experienced diabetic ketoacidosis and hyperglycemia. However, these trials emphasize the necessity of assessing autoantibody status in addition to thyroid function and fasting hyperglycemia before starting IL-2 therapy. When an autoimmune endocrinopathy develops, diet is a major factor. Autoimmune diabetes is frequently linked to dietary components like carbohydrates and fatty acids, while autoimmune thyroid disorders are mostly influenced by the vitamin iodine. One of the primary causes of dysregulated glucose metabolism and obesity has been identified as nutritional toxicity, or the overconsumption of foods with high nutritional values. As a result, the course of several autoimmune endocrinopathies is determined by behavioral and dietary factors. Over the past ten years, there has been an increase in the incidence of obesity in the US, which raises the risk of diabetes. Obesity is caused by a sedentary lifestyle and consuming large meals that are high in fatty acids, fiber, cholesterol, and added sugars. Type 2 diabetes, dyslipidemia, hypertension, and impaired glucose tolerance are frequently accompanied by obesity. Age, sex, and the geographic distribution affect eating habits. Few studies have established a direct correlation between nutrition and type 1 diabetes, even though diet plays an important role in the development of endocrinopathies. A significant association was found between the effects of a modified high-fat diet on regulated insulin-like growth factor (IGF) and IGF-binding protein in a comprehensive study comparing the effects of dietary changes among Indians who had moved to the UK and those who had not.

7.12 Diet components

It has been demonstrated that elevated glucose and fatty acid levels both overstimulate beta-pancreatic cells, impairing their ability to function. Although a direct effect of hypersensitivity has been noted, very little is known about the immune-mediated effects brought on by excessive glucose ingestion. There are research studies that explain how fatty acids affect autoimmune diabetes. Obesity and poor glucose tolerance were linked in studies using transgenic mice with decreased muscle insulin receptor signaling. Only fatty acids belonging to the Omega 3 family have been demonstrated to be protective against glucose intolerance. The NF-kB signaling pathway, which is driven by cytokines like IL-1 and IFN-γ, is one of the pathways proposed for fatty acid-induced beta-cell death(Donath et al., 2003). Fas expression, beta-cell death, and NO generation follow the start of NF-kB signaling. The fatty acids and cytokines may trigger beta-cell death through other processes that are not dependent on NF-kB signaling. NF-kB activation has also been shown to play a protective function in cytokine-mediated beta-cell death. It is evident that the immune system plays an important role in the death of pancreatic beta-cells brought on by excessive fatty acid exposure; however, there may be other underlying mechanisms. Iodine has been identified as a key dietary component that contributes to the development of hypothyroidism and hyperthyroidism. Disease is due to the interaction of genetic, hormonal, and environmental variables. National policies pertaining to iodine supplementation in meals were influenced by epidemiological research that demonstrated a substantial correlation between thyroid dysfunction and iodine deficiency. The 1920s saw the introduction of iodination of salt as a public health precaution. Due to the program's great success, endemic goiter in the US was essentially eradicated. However, the steadily rising dietary iodine concentration was accompanied by an increase in the incidence of autoimmune thyroiditis. For instance, when iodine deficiency was eradicated in a region of endemic goiter in northwest Greece, the prevalence of autoimmune thyroiditis among schoolchildren increased threefold. Thyroiditis in genetically predisposed individuals is linked to this higher iodine intake. Among the sources of dietary iodine include foods and food additives, topical antiseptics, and drugs.

After being given iodine again, some patients with reversed hypothyroidism developed hypothyroidism again. Iodine restriction helped many patients with primary hypothyroidism regain normal thyroid function. Therefore, autoimmune thyroid disease can be induced by high iodine consumption, but only in those who are genetically predisposed. The thyroid follicular cells, which store iodides, contain a large protein called the Tg molecule. Tyrosines make up 67 of the 2748 amino acids that make up each human Tg chain. Iodination occurs in 25% of tyrosines(Burek & Rose, 2008). It is believed that just four of the tyrosines in each chain are involved in hormonogenesis. The four hormonogenic tyrosyl sites are not the only ones that can be used to store iodine. Tg becomes more stable and resistant to proteolysis when iodine binds more strongly to tyrosyl residues. Human studies reveal that when Tg was depleted of iodine, both antibody and in vitro T-cell responses returned to reference levels. These responses were recovered by thyroglobulin re-iodination. Monoclonal antibodies have shown that changing the iodine concentration of human Tg can both produce new epitopes and make others inaccessible. Since conducting in-depth study on human subjects is challenging, animal models have been used for the majority of the studies. Since non-iodinated Tg is unable to generate severe thyroiditis, iodine-containing epitopes play a significant role in the induction of thyroid autoimmunity. These results imply that T-cell identification may be the starting point for iodine action. Research conducted on animal models has conclusively demonstrated that iodine plays a destructive role in autoimmune thyroid disease. Animal studies have consistently shown that a higher dietary iodine intake causes the disease to develop earlier and more severely. The disease only affects a subset of genetically predisposed animals. A high-iodine diet boosts the immune responses to Tg. Iodine restriction delays lymphocytic infiltration. In the iodine-enhanced NOD, thyroiditis must be initiated by both CD4 and CD8 T cells. In a H2H4 model; however, only CD4 cells are needed to sustain the disease chronicity, since CD8 cell depletion decreased disease severity but not CD4 cell depletion, indicating that CD8 cells are not required to sustain the progression to severe thyroiditis. It has also been shown that B lymphocytes, particularly in the early stages of life, were necessary for the development of NOD disease. After using an anti-IgM therapy to decrease B cells, researchers discovered that thyroiditis worsened. Thyroiditis was not brought on by passive antibody transfer or adult B cell reconstitution, indicating that B cells were necessary and that they play a significant role in antigen presentation. Although THs and other iodinated compounds are known to play a role in the transition of monocytes to dendritic cells mediated by components like granulocyte-monocyte colony-stimulating factor (GM-CSF), TNF-α, and IL-6, and are demonstrated to significantly affect the immune responses, there is less evidence for the effects of differentially iodinated Tg on the function of antigen presenting cells (APCs). Iodine may therefore directly modify APCs to start the process that results in thyroiditis. These findings also imply that the critical events that lead to the development of diseases are different from those that occur during the chronic stage. Even after stopping excess iodine, there is no discernible decrease in disease once it has been established, indicating that the early triggers are particularly crucial in influencing how the disease develops in the future.

7.13 ICAM-1

Iodine causes Intercellular adhesion molecule-1 (ICAM-1) to be upregulated initially, which advances thyroid disease. ICAM-1 is constitutively expressed by NOD.H2h4 mice thyrocytes, and its expression is significantly increased after a few weeks of iodine feeding(Bonita et al., 2002). Within 24 hours of iodine stimulation, an increase in ICAM-1 expression was seen. Iodine alone may therefore promote elevated ICAM-1 expression, which explains the initial stimulation in disease. It has been demonstrated that ICAM-1 is crucial for identifying the location of inflammatory mononuclear cells in the early phases of inflammatory immune responses. Increased ICAM-1 expression in the thyroid glands of patients with Graves' disease and Hashimoto's thyroiditis has also been documented in many comparable human studies. Researchers have extended these findings to comprehend the mechanisms of ICAM-1 regulation using the NOD.H2h4 mouse model. At least three distinct transcriptional start sites and many transcription binding sites are present in the ICAM-1 gene promoter. Many stimuli, including specific cytokines, viruses, radiation, retinoic acid, and oxidants, can increase the expression of ICAM-1. Through the thyroperoxidase enzyme reaction, iodine is absorbed by the thyrocyte, and stored on the Tg molecule. Reactive oxygen species (ROS) such as hydrogen peroxide and superoxide anion are produced during this process. The ICAM-1 gene promoter is known to be stimulated by both of these ROS. This process is initiated in genetically predisposed individuals by a variety of minor stressors, resulting in an overexpression of ICAM-1 in the thyroid gland. In animals, ICAM-1 expression in iodine-treated thyrocytes was decreased in vitro by ROS blocking with specific pharmacological inhibitors. Since the cultures lacked immune cells, the elevated ICAM-1 was only caused by iodine. Iodine can have both direct and indirect effects on thyrocytes through the production of cytokines by invading lymphocytes.

7.14 Smoking

Smoking cigarettes is a serious public health issue and is linked to type 1 diabetes. Few studies have directly demonstrated that the condition is autoimmune, and none have identified the immunogenic effects of smoke on the onset of disease. It was discovered that there was a considerable dose-dependent increase in cICAM-1 levels. Some studies discovered that T1DM patients who smoked had higher levels of endothelium ICAM (ECAM)-1 and vascular ICAM (VCAM)-1. Although the precise mechanism causing smoking-induced type 1 diabetes is unknown, elevated plasma levels of cICAM-1 and cVCAM-1 raise the possibility that one mechanism of beta-cell death is increased inflammation, cell-cell contact, and inflammatory cytokine release. It is challenging to determine whether the disease is autoimmune in the absence of any antibody data. Graves' disease with ophthalmopathy, and different types of hyperthyroidism and hypothyroidism were examined. Among current smokers, a dose-response association between rising disease risk was reported. There was a high correlation between smoking patients and Graves' disease with ophthalmopathy. There was a significant correlation between Graves' disease and current smokers as opposed to ex-smokers. Women smokers had a higher correlation with Graves' disease There are few research studies on the relationship between smoking and subclinical hypothyroidism. Thyroid peroxidase antibodies were found to be less common in women in the Netherlands. It was discovered that smokers and thyroid autoimmunity were negatively correlated. The mechanisms underlying thyroid disorders brought on by cigarette smoking are mostly unknown. Thyroid gland function may be impacted by thiocyanate, a chemical produced by smoking, according to some studies. Iodine-trapping mechanisms are known to be inhibited by thiocyanate and perchlorate ions.

7.15 Breastfeeding and diabetes

Breastfeeding has a minor protective effect on infants with type 1 diabetes, while formula diets have some negative consequences. Similarly, there were no discernible negative effects on islet cell autoimmunity from the early introduction of cow milk and dairy products. There was no correlation between the length of time spent breastfeeding or drinking cow milk and islet cell autoimmunity in research involving children who developed type 1 diabetes. It was discovered that children with higher genetic susceptibility (HLA-DQB1) were more likely to develop beta-cell autoimmunity following early cow's milk introduction or short-term breastfeeding. Nutrition can affect how infants with the HLA-DQB1 genotype manipulate their spontaneous beta-cell autoimmunity(Åkerblom et al., 2005). It is difficult to draw conclusions on the relationship between autoimmune diabetes and newborn dietary variables based on the majority of human studies. The thyroid health of newborns is significantly impacted by decreased breastfeeding patterns brought on by high work demands and changing lifestyles. Many formula feeds in different combinations are frequently used in place of breastfeeding, which has increased the risk of thyroid autoimmune disease in babies. Additional studies have looked into how giving cow's milk and newborn formula affects kids' health. Known for being a competitive inhibitor of the sodium iodide transporter, perchlorate is a goitrogenic anion that is frequently found in cow's milk across the US. Nearly 80% of perchlorate is metabolized in the lumen and may pose a risk to cattle. The remaining percentage that comes from cow's milk may also cause goiter in babies and damage their thyroid and neurological development. The general health of occupational workers exposed to perchlorate for an average of 1.7 years was not significantly impacted. Serum TSH and Tg concentrations did not show any discernible increases, but serum T4, free T4, and free T3 concentrations, however marginally higher than controls, were significant. Breastfeeding has been shown to provide long-lasting protective benefits.

7.16 Autoimmune disease and industrial waste

Autoimmune thyroid disease has been linked to exposure to industrial wastes such hexachlorobenzene, polychlorinated biphenyls, and organochlorine insecticides like thiocyanate and perchlorates. Workers exposed to polychlorinated biphenyls had elevated TSH, reduced T4, and anti-thyroid antibodies. There is evidence linking exposure to dithiocarbamates and ethylenebisdithiocarbamate to increased thyroid size and other thyroid-related abnormalities. The effects of perchlorate and thiocyanate on thyroid function were investigated in a longitudinal study of occupational workers in an ammonia production plant. At the sodium-iodide symporter level, these substances are directly linked to iodine uptake in the thyroid. The workers who were exposed for three days (12 hours each day) had somewhat higher levels of serum T4, free T4, and total T3 than workers who were not exposed for three days(El-Benhawy et al., 2022). In addition to age, sex, and genetics that change disease pathology, it is crucial to take into account the severity and length of exposure. Chemicals immediately start and worsen the pathogenic immunological process, mutate genes, change regulatory and immune effector pathways, and alter immune tolerance. Sometimes, systemic allergic reactions mimic autoimmune-like symptoms and develop into autoimmune diseases. In autoimmune processes, the immune system reacts to the autoantigens, but in systemic allergic reactions, the immune system may react to the chemical molecule. Chemicals or xenobiotics can change how the thyroid gland functions directly by changing the structure of the thyroid or indirectly by changing how regulatory enzymes that are engaged at different stages of TH synthesis work. The thyroid gland produces THs T3 and T4, which are then released into the bloodstream and delivered to various tissues. TH production is impacted by chemicals like thiocyanate and perchlorate, which block iodine uptake at the symporter level or during thyrotropin stimulation.

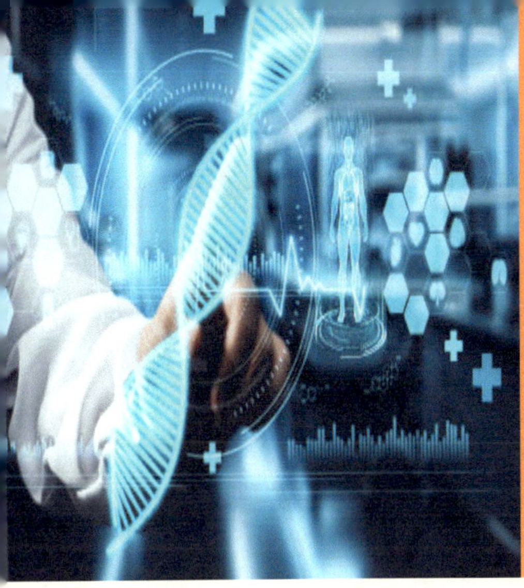

Chapter 8
GENOMICS

Contents

8.1 Introduction

The underlying origin of the systemic, chronic inflammatory disease known as rheumatoid arthritis (RA) is unknown. With an estimated 1% frequency in adults, it is the most prevalent type of inflammatory arthritis. With a female : male ratio of 2.5:1, women are more likely than men to get the disease(Geraghty et al., 2021). Although the disease can attack at any age, the 40s are the peak age at which it first manifests, and the incidence rises with age. Significant clinical variability exists, as is the case with many complicated diseases that are influenced by several genes and environmental factors.

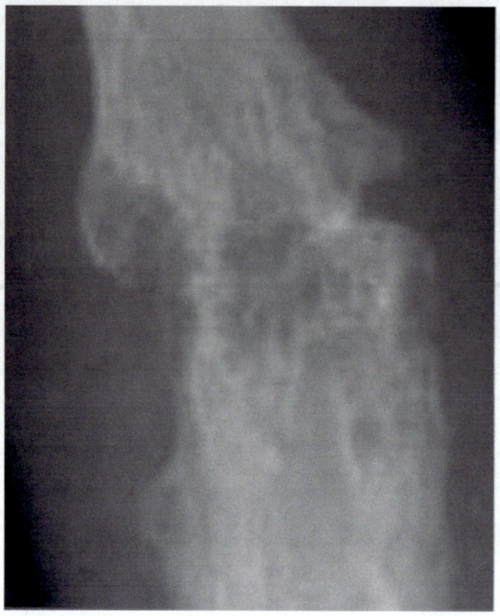

Figure 8.1 Articular erosions

Source: https://upload.wikimedia.org/wikipedia/commons/6/6c/X-ray_of_right_fourth_PIP_joint_with_bone_erosions_by_rheumatoid_arthritis.jpg,*Creative Commons License.*

Articular erosions (Figure 8.1) and joint abnormalities (Figure 8.2) arise with chronic disease.

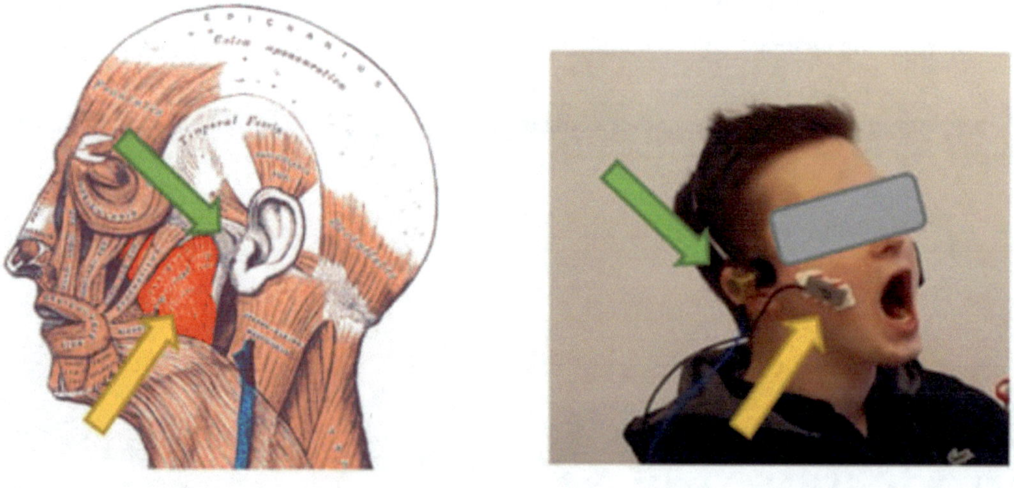

Figure 8.2 Joint abnormalities

Source: Kulesa-Mrowiecka, M., Barański, R., & Kłaczyński, M. (2022). sEMG and Vibration System Monitoring for Differential Diagnosis in Temporomandibular Joint Disorders. Sensors, 22(10), 3811. https://doi.org/10.3390/s22103811,*Creative Commons License.*

Autoantibodies have been used in the clinical management of RA and have significant diagnostic properties. Gene studies of disease susceptibility have been the main focus of research to comprehend the molecular basis of RA. Only two genes, PTPN22 and HLA-DRB1, have been shown to significantly affect the risk of RA, and only a limited portion of the genome has been examined using the molecular genetic techniques currently in use. Although they are less developed, other genomic methods including large-scale expression and proteome profiling in RA are good for comprehending the etiology of the disease. The clinical management of RA patients has been largely unaffected by genomic medicine, which translates genomic information into predictions of disease susceptibility, characterization of gene - environment interactions, identification of new therapeutic targets, and development of novel gene-based diagnostics. Despite being recognized since the 1970s, the link between HLA-DRB1 allele susceptibility has not resulted in any innovative diagnostic or therapy approaches. The creation of inhibitors of tumor necrosis factor-alpha (TNF-α), a crucial cytokine, is an achievement in the therapeutic management of RA that resulted from extensive research. The goal of genomic medicine advancements is to improve patient care for this disease by matching the effectiveness of TNF inhibitors.

8.2 RA and MHC

The underlying cause of RA remains unknown despite decades of investigation. Although just two genes (PTPN22 and HLA-DRB1) and one environmental factor (smoking) have been linked to RA susceptibility in several studies, genes and environment work together to contribute to the development of RA. Anti-CCP antibodies, which are antibodies against cyclic citrullinated peptides, have become a specific indicator for RA. The fact that anti-CCP antibodies exist years before RA is diagnosed implies that these autoantibodies are harmful rather than merely a sign of persistent inflammation. These risk factors point to a framework in which an environmental trigger, such as smoking, causes genetically susceptible hosts to mount an immune response, resulting in the development of autoantibodies and ultimately RA. Family studies and genome-wide linkage studies have shown the genetic component of RA susceptibility in humans. The degree of phenotypic variation brought about by additive genetic factors as opposed to common environmental influences, random variation, gene-environment interactions, and gene-gene interactions is known as heritability. Approximately 60% of disease variability is inherited. Comparing the prevalence of disease in family members to the general population provides another indicator of the genetic contribution to disease activity. A patient monozygotic (MZ) twin had a 15% risk of developing RA, compared to 1% for the general population. The number varies depending on the population investigated, but for RA, the relative risk (RR) to the sibling of a proband with RA is 5. On the short arm of human chromosome 6, the major histocompatibility complex (MHC) region covers 3.6 megabases (Mb) and has hundreds of genes, many of which are involved in immunological function. An estimated one-third of the total genetic component of RA risk is thought to be accounted for by the MHC region of the human genome. This region has been frequently identified as significant in the pathophysiology of RA by genome-wide linkage scans employing both single nucleotide polymorphism (SNP) markers and microsatellites (Yamamoto & Yamada, 2005). The MHC area has the highest genetic contribution in RA, according to these genome-wide scans, and the relative contribution of MHC genes (MHC) was determined to be 1.75. Alleles in the HLA-DRB1 gene are linked to a large portion, but most likely not all, of the risk attributed to the MHC region. The mixed lymphocyte culture (MCL) type Dw4, which is connected to the serological subtype DR4, was found to be more prevalent in RA patients than in controls in the 1970s, marking the first evidence of a connection between RA and the Class II HLA proteins. The serological Dw4 subtype was then identified as belonging to the HLA-DRB1 gene by examining the molecular variation of Class II proteins. Some researchers observed a common amino acid sequence at positions 70 -74 of the HLA-DRB1 protein. Since these residues are crucial for peptide binding, it was postulated that RA-associated alleles bind certain peptides, hence promoting the growth of auto-reactive T cells.

MHC Class II molecules contain a protein that is encoded by the HLA-DRB1 gene. The antigen presenting cells (APCs) contain these molecules, which are heterodimers of alpha and beta proteins. They show CD4 T cells (T helper) peptides produced from external proteins. The MHC region has some subregions that are 1 Mb and contain the genes encoding the Class II molecules. Three beta-chain genes and one alpha-chain gene have been identified within the DR subregion; the a-chain gene and two beta-chain genes, DRB1 and DRB2, are both highly expressed. DX and DQ-alpha and beta are two sets of alpha and beta-chain genes found in the DQ subregion. Significant allelic diversity is seen in all of the expressed genes, except for DR-alpha.

8.3 HLA alleles

Many population studies have confirmed the link between RA and allelic variations at HLA-DRB1. Different DRB1 alleles have varying degrees of genetic link with RA susceptibility, even though HLA-DRB1 susceptibility alleles are frequently regarded as a group. HLA-DRB1 risk alleles fall into at least two classes: high and moderate. A protective allele may be in linkage disequilibrium with the HLA-DRB1 alleles. Once the impact of the shared epitope alleles has been taken into account, it has been hypothesized that the presence of an asparagine amino acid at position 70 of the HLA-DRB1 protein (D70) may be linked to protection against the development of RA. HLA-DRB1 susceptibility alleles affect the severity of chronic diseases, especially when it comes to the emergence of bony erosions(Pyeritz, 2023). The existence of CCP autoantibodies is the main cause of this association. Whether HLA-DRB1 alleles increase the risk of erosive disease without being influenced by CCP autoantibodies is still unknown. The fact that certain investigations have shown that SE alleles predict erosive variations, but only in RF patients, may be explained by this finding. Since SE alleles are known to have a higher correlation with CCP than RF/RA, one theory to explain this observation is that RF patients in these earlier investigations are actually CCP. It will be crucial to evaluate the association between HLA-DRB1 alleles and clinical outcomes in the future, accounting for the impact of CCP and other significant clinical factors. The exact mechanism by which the HLA-DRB1 alleles contribute to the risk of RA remains unclear after decades of research.

The SE alleles are thought to influence T-cell activation thresholds, thymic selection of high-affinity self-reactive T cells, and molecular mimicry of microbial antigens. It is important to note that the third hypervariable region of the protein has a peptide-binding groove that presents peptides to CD4 T cells. In HLA-DRB1 *0401 transgenic mice, citrullination of specific peptides results in a robust immune response to citrullinated peptides(Sakkas et al., 2014). After accounting for the impact of HLADRB1, many studies indicate that other genes within the MHC probably contribute to disease susceptibility. RA may be linked to an extended haplotype that contains HLA-DRB1 DR3 alleles. Class III MHC genes, including the TNF-alpha region mentioned in some studies, are present in the 500 kb linked haplotype. According to some studies, this link only applies to patients with CCP. No single study has thoroughly examined MHC DNA variants in a patient group enough to identify effects other than HLA-DRB1 alleles. The concept that non-HLA-DRB1 alleles affect the likelihood of having RA has only recently been tested with the availability of genetic linkage disequilibrium maps. The use of high-density SNP genotyping (Figure 8.3) in patient groups ought to shed more light on how the MHC region affects RA severity and susceptibility. It has been difficult to identify the genes causing RA that are not located in the MHC region. According to some research studies, these non-HLA genes account for up to two-thirds of genetic diversity. T-cell activation threshold is influenced by PTPN22, the gene with the strong replication.

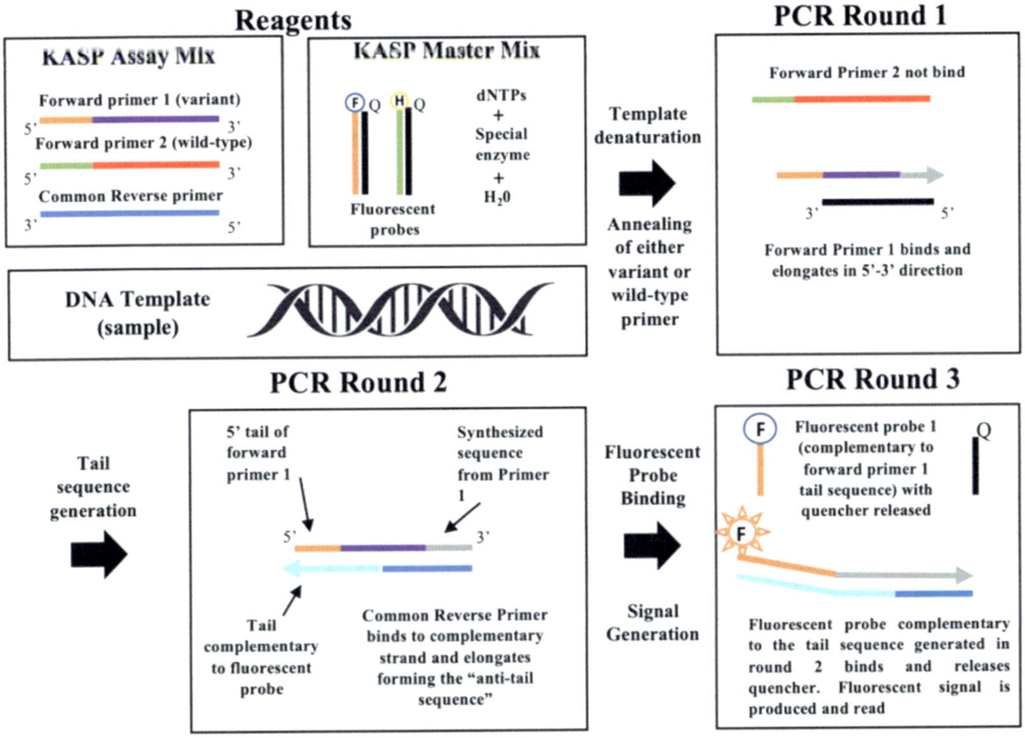

Figure 8.3 SNP genotyping

Source: Lawrie, R. D., & Massey, S. E. (2023). Agrigenomic Diversity Unleashed: Current Single Nucleotide Polymorphism Genotyping Methods for the Agricultural Sciences. Applied Biosciences, 2(4), 565-585. https://doi.org/10.3390/applbiosci2040036,*Creative Commons License.*

8.4 Other alleles

It has been confirmed by many studies that PTPN22 is the non-HLA gene linked to RA. T-cell activation is altered by the susceptibility allele, a missense mutation that converts an arginine to tryptophan amino acid (R620W). The OR indicates that the genetic influence is comparable to other SE alleles, although it is significantly smaller than that of HLA-DRB1*0401. This genotype is not linked to susceptibility in Japanese populations because it is lacking in East Asians. Unlike HLA-DRB1, PTPN22 has not been the subject of extensive genotype-phenotype associations. Similar to HLA-DRB1 alleles, PTPN22 is only linked to seropositive RA. There is no evidence that PTPN22 affects disease activity or radiographic erosions, but there is some evidence that it influences the age of onset of disease and may have a significant effect in males than females. Other genes have been linked to RA in genetic association studies, but they have not yet attained the statistical significance needed to be confirmed as actual RA-susceptibility genes. Among the potential genes are SLC22A4, PADI4, and CTLA4. Type 1 diabetes and autoimmune thyroiditis provide the evidence linking CTLA4 polymorphisms to autoimmunity susceptibility. T-cell activation is negatively regulated by CTLA4. An allele in the gene 3 untranslated region (UTR) raises the likelihood of developing these conditions. These results have been extended to RA by several investigations, where the genetic influence is small. PADI4 may play a significant role in the production of anti-CCP autoantibodies since it encodes an enzyme that post-translationally converts arginine to citrulline. A mutation was linked to disease risk in an initial report in Japanese patients. Although subsequent results have been less statistically compelling, they nevertheless show a connection with RA susceptibility. Some researchers suggested that a common allele within the SLC22A4 gene may be linked to RA susceptibility among East Asian populations; however, other researchers found no evidence of this association in RA patients of European lineage. Hematological and immunological tissues produce the organic cation transporter protein product of SLC22A4(Ciarimboli, 2016). RA patients with European lineage have a lower population frequency of the putative causal allele, which disrupts an RUNX1-binding site, than patients with East Asian lineage. This limits the ability to identify an association in RA patients with European lineage.

Only a small portion of the human genome genetic variation has been examined in the majority of studies conducted to date. Although the human genome is thought to contain approximately 10 million common variants, only a negligible portion of these variants are tested in the majority of research. The majority of disease alleles have a relatively low anticipated genetic effect. As a result, thousands of patients are needed to identify the genetic effect, and the majority of research has only been done on a smaller number of patients, which limits the ability to identify an actual positive association. RA and other autoimmune disorders will be the subject of genome-wide association studies, which examine the majority of prevalent genetic variations in the human genome. These investigations should significantly increase the list of RA-susceptibility genes if they are properly analyzed. With genotyping systems that capture around 60% of common genetic variations, several genome-wide association studies are now in progress.

8.5 RA and other factors

Women are more than twice as likely as men to get RA, and this difference is even more pronounced at a younger age. This makes females possibly the strongest non-genetic risk factor for the development of RA. The chance of having RA in women rises with age and peaks around menopause. Due to these findings, a lot of work has been done to investigate how hormones and pregnancy-related factors affect the development of disease. RA symptoms are less severe during the post-ovulatory phase of the menstrual cycle and during pregnancy, and the risk of developing RA increases during the 12-month postpartum period.

The time spent breastfeeding may be linked to an increased risk of RA. The risk of having

RA is doubled for women who breastfeed for 24 months in total. Serum testosterone levels in RA patients are consistently lower, according to cross-sectional investigations of serum androgen levels(Tuin et al., 2013).

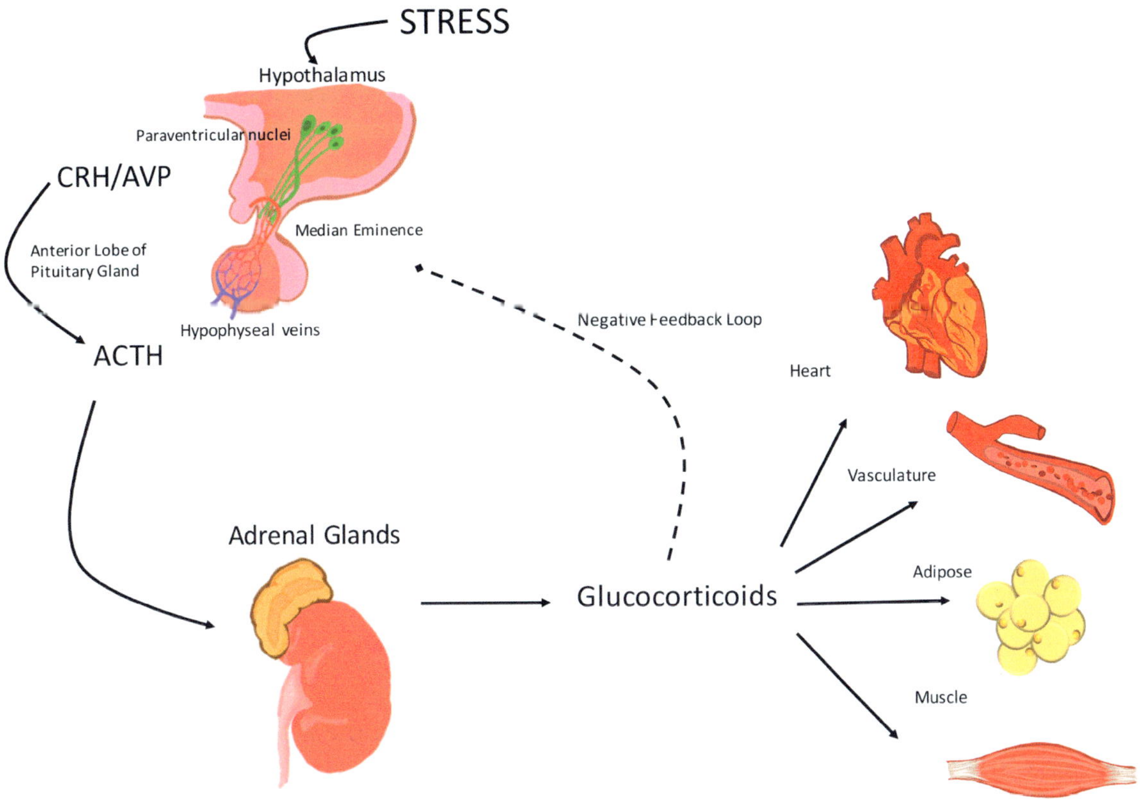

Figure 8.4 Hypothalamic-pituitary axis

Source: Burford, N. G., Webster, N. A., & Cruz-Topete, D. (2017). Hypothalamic-Pituitary-Adrenal Axis Modulation of Glucocorticoids in the Cardiovascular System. International Journal of Molecular Sciences, 18(10), 2150. https://doi.org/10.3390/ijms18102150,*Creative Commons License.*

Patients with RA have changes in the hypothalamic-pituitary axis (HPA) (Figure 8.4), and RA is linked to diseases that cause hypoadrenalism and panhypopituitarism. In accordance with the function of estrogen in humans, castration of female mice exacerbates arthritis, and estrogen replacement therapy reduces arthritis in the collagen-induced mouse model of arthritis and adjuvant arthritis in rats. Some RA patients experience remarkable remission when pregnant. This phenomenon has been explained by fetal-maternal genetic relationships, but other evidence contradicts this theory. It is likely that hormonal changes during pregnancy account for at least some of the disease remission during pregnancy. Although genes within steroid hormone pathways have been suggested to play a role in the hereditary risk of RA, no gene has been definitively identified as of yet. The environmental risk factor strongly linked to the development of RA is smoking. Many studies conducted over the past 20 years have conclusively demonstrated that smoking raises the chance of developing RA by a factor of 2.0 for both males and females. The majority of these studies show that heavy, current smokers have the highest chance of developing autoantibody-positive RA; nevertheless, the risk persists for around ten years after quitting smoking. Some researchers examined the risk of developing disease in carriers of these risk factors because the association between smoking and autoantibody-positive RA is similar to the genetic association between HLA-DRB1 alleles and autoantibody-positive RA. They found that smokers with two copies of the SE alleles had a 16-fold increased risk of developing RF-RA. Blood transfusions, obesity, occupational exposure to silica and mineral oils, and socioeconomic status are additional potential environmental risk factors that have not been as extensively studied as smoking. Several of these environmental agents are inhaled through the lungs. Similar to cigarette smoke exposure, silica dust, and mineral oil exposure were risk factors exclusively for seropositive RA. Mineral oil can be used as an adjuvant to cause experimental arthritis in mouse models. Although there is indirect evidence, it is by no means definitive that exposure to an infectious agent or agents may cause RA. However, no specific infectious agent has been identified as a risk factor for RA.

In the diagnosis and prognosis of RA patients, autoantibodies are useful. About two-thirds of RA patients have autoantibodies, which indicate advanced disease. Anti-cyclic citrullinated peptide (CCP) antibodies, which are antibodies against peptides with arginine post-translationally modified to citrulline, and RF, an immunoglobulin specific to the Fc region of IgG, are the two main types of autoantibodies used clinically to generate RA subsets. Despite their high correlation, these autoantibodies might be different clinical subgroups of RA. One of the diagnostic criteria for RA is the presence of RF autoantibodies. However, due to its low sensitivity and specificity, the RF assay is still not the best diagnostic tool available. Anti-CCP antibodies predict radiographic erosions in patients with early-onset RA and have a moderate sensitivity but an elevated specificity for RA. The question of whether these autoantibodies are a non-specific reaction to systemic inflammation or if they are causative has been debated. There is significant clinical heterogeneity, just like in other complicated human diseases. RF and CCP antibodies have been utilized to select patients in the search for RA genes since their presence or absence offers a logical clinical subgroup. HLA-DRB1 and PTPN22, two genes that are clearly linked to RA, are in fact linked to CCP patients but not CCP patients (Conigliaro et al., 2016).

8.6 Speculations

It is interesting to speculate about a potential model of RA pathogenesis. Smoking or other air pollutants lead to inflammation and citrullination of proteins in the lungs in genetically sensitive individuals. Anti-CCP antibodies are produced as a result of this process, and they directly cause disease in the joint. HLA-DRB1 variations enhance the autoimmune response, and citrullinated proteins are shown in class II MHC molecules to elicit an immune response. The PTPN22 missense mutation might increase the autoimmune response or enable autoreactive T-cells to evade thymus selection. Even if certain parts of this model might be accurate, it most likely does not account for the pathophysiology of RA in every patient. Clinical research must continue to be integrated to refine models of RA pathogenesis. The development of genome-wide association studies should make it easier to find additional genes linked to RA and advance our knowledge of the pathophysiology of the disease. Although neither has been extensively used in large patient samples, other genetic resources are available to examine the susceptibility to RA, such as mRNA expression profiling and serum protein level analysis. The availability of affordable, high-throughput assays continues to be a constraint on the proteomics field. It has also proven difficult to find auto-antigens that predispose to RA. These initiatives aim to find new biomarkers that could be used as therapeutic targets or that enable early and precise disease diagnosis or predict severe disease. The effectiveness of RF and anti-CCP autoantibodies shows that a new biomarker may be directly useful in therapeutic settings. Genome-wide study of mRNA expression patterns has been performed in peripheral blood and synovial fluid obtained from RA patients. This method has proven useful in the peripheral blood of individuals with systemic lupus erythematosus (SLE). Studies in peripheral blood have compared RA patients to normal controls, RF versus RF patients, and early versus chronic RA. Comparing inflammatory RA synovium to non-inflammatory OA synovium in synovial tissue has been done using similar methods.

8.7 The role of cytokines

Through the effective investigation of hundreds of thousands of genes for influences on disease risk, genome-wide genetic association studies and mRNA expression profiling enable the investigations. These systems are becoming more reliable and affordable.

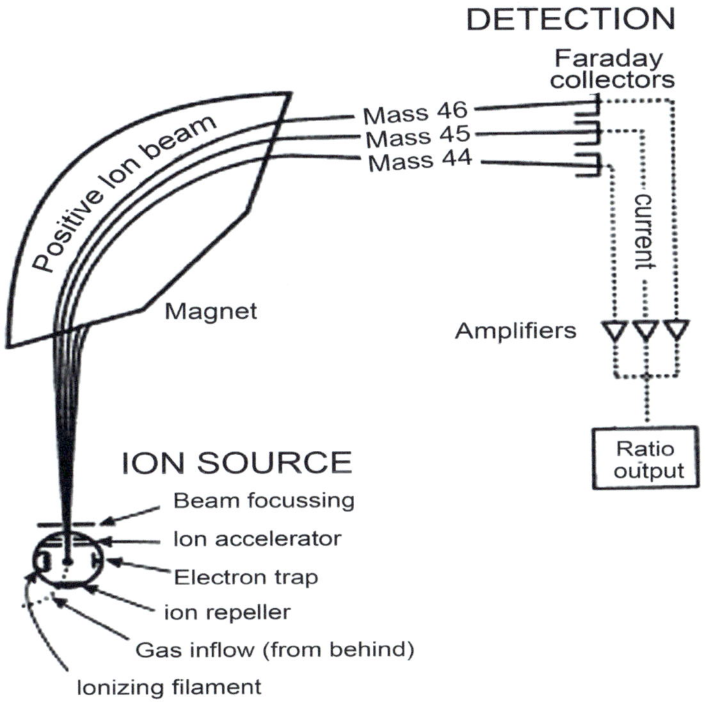

Figure 8.5 Mass spectrometry

Source: https://upload.wikimedia.org/wikipedia/commons/b/b8/Mass_spectrometer_schematics.png,*Creative Commons License.*

Proteomics, on the other hand, has faced comparable technical challenges. Although it provides such a platform, mass spectrometry is not yet extensively utilized. Because ELISA-based techniques cannot do high-throughput multiplexing, the majority of proteomics research in RA and other complicated diseases has been restricted to a small number of proteins of significance. It is evident that cytokines are essential to the pathophysiology of RA. Within the immune system, cytokines are soluble proteins that facilitate intercellular communication. Important examples include the proinflammatory cytokines tumor necrosis factor-alpha (TNF-alpha) and interleukin 1 (IL1), together with their soluble receptors(Steeve et al., 2004). Macrophages in the synovium are the main source of these cytokines, which cause inflammation and stimulation of synovial tissue effector functions such as cellular proliferation, metalloproteinase and adhesion-molecule production, and prostaglandin and other cytokine secretion. Neutralizing therapies that target the proteins themselves in patients with active RA may provide the evidence for the role of cytokines in RA pathogenesis. Antibodies against TNF-α have proven remarkably helpful in the treatment of RA, while anti-IL1 therapies are somewhat effective but not as effective as anti-TNF-α therapies. Although cytokines play a significant role in RA, it is unclear if changes in cytokine secretion cause RA or if dysfunction is just the outcome of an overreactive immune system. The evidence required to establish causality has not yet been found in any longitudinal investigations that show changes in these molecules before the onset of RA. An alternative method of proving causation would be to show that RA develops as a result of genetic variation within a cytokine gene. Although many studies have indicated that TNF gene alleles affect the risk of RA, it has not yet been demonstrated that this effect is unaffected by linkage disequilibrium with HLA-DRB1 or nearby genes in the 3.6 Mb MHC area. Theoretically, every allele influencing a particular cytokine release could be mapped and subsequently examined to see if they also affect the onset of RA.

8.8 Techniques for cytokine analysis in RA

It is important to highlight research that has used multiplex cytokine arrays, mass spectrometry (Figure 8.5), and antigen microarrays to examine synovial fluid and serum in RA patients. A two-step mass spectrometry method was employed to produce protein profiles of synovial fluid from individuals with either erosive or non-erosive RA. C-reactive protein (CRP) and six calcium-binding protein members of the S100 protein family were among the 33 proteins that were found to be higher in the synovial fluid of patients with erosive RA. Patients with erosive RA also had higher serum levels of the proteins S100A8 (calgranulin A), S100A12 (calgranulin C), and CRP. One of the five proteins found to be elevated in the serum of patients with CCP RA was hypothesized to be myeloid-related protein 8 (MRP8). Patients with RA may have higher levels of the MRP8 protein in their synovial fluid than those with osteoarthritis. Autoantibody reactivity against citrullinated epitopes is more prevalent in patients with elevated serum levels of TNF, IL-15, IL-1, IL-6, IL-13, and GM-CSF(Serre, 2001). They demonstrated this using microarray in a group of early RA patients. There are currently no effective ways to test for RA in a population before the disease manifests. Together with genetic susceptibility variations, the existence of CCP autoantibodies may significantly raise the risk to the point where screening the healthy population is economical. Since RA treatments presently focus on symptoms rather than a cure, it is unclear whether an effective intervention to prevent

RA will arise under these circumstances. One-third of RA patients who develop autoantibody-negative disease are not screened by this simple method. Although they cannot predict a patient's prognosis on their own, the degree of synovial inflammation and the presence of autoantibodies at the time of initial diagnosis indicate a bad prognosis. Likewise, whereas HLA-DRB1 SE alleles indicate more severe disease, they are not frequently taken into consideration when making clinical patient care decisions. The prognosis of an untreated patient is more influenced by responsiveness to treatment than by the severity of the underlying disease because treatment approaches have significantly improved over the past ten years with the introduction of TNF-α treatment.

8.9 Treatment of RA

Early initiation of disease-modifying medications, or DMARDs, is a primary objective of treatment. Weekly low doses of methotrexate (MTX) are the most widely used disease-modifying treatment. This medication can be used alone, in conjunction with biologic response modifiers, or in combination with other synthetic compounds such as sulfasalazine, or antimalarials. One significant development in RA treatment has been the development of biologics that block the pro-inflammatory cytokine TNF-α. In addition to improving quality of life and slowing the rate of radiographic progression, monoclonal antibodies and the p75 TNF-α soluble receptor fusion protein can be used alone or in conjunction with MTX to reduce disease signs and symptoms. When used with MTX, these treatments work well. Rituximab, a B-cell depleting technique, and abatacept, which blocks the CTLA4 co-stimulation pathway, are two more recent biologics that have been licensed for treatment in RA. This disease has been significantly impacted by early MTX intervention and combination therapy, which includes anti-TNF-α therapy.

8.10 Mapping associations with multiple sclerosis

Association mapping searches for genetic markers that are more prevalent in MS patients than in controls, and indicates a connection between an allelic variation and a disease phenotype. Although the MHC locus has been associated with genetic susceptibility to multiple sclerosis, the specific gene or genes responsible for this susceptibility are not clear, especially in light of the pattern of linkage disequilibrium seen for this chromosomal site. Therefore, in addition to HLA-DRB1, other genes within the MHC locus may also be linked to MS; TNF and other loci in HLA class III and HLA class I are candidates. To determine the gene or genes in the MHC region causing the elevated susceptibility to MS, some researchers used a high-density SNP panel to genotype some patients from Finland and Canada. According to their findings, the DRB1 allele in the HLA class II region is the only significant susceptibility locus in the MHC region; however, the real susceptibility variant may still be present in a nearby locus. Consequently, the MS susceptibility to the roughly 100 kb stretch flanking HLA-DRB1 was confirmed by association mapping. On the one hand, this study shows how association has more strength than linkage mapping. However, it also emphasizes how association mapping is dependent on linkage disequilibrium.

Admixture mapping is an association mapping technique predicated on two factors. They are a disparity in disease prevalence between two ethnic groups and the presence of a third admixed population. Northern Europeans and Africans are less susceptible to a variety of autoimmune, circulatory, and metabolic diseases, including multiple sclerosis(Koriem, 2016). In North America, where MS is more common among European Americans than

African Americans, this differential susceptibility is also seen. There has not been much chromosomal recombination between African and European lineage in the history of African American communities since, on average, only six generations have passed since African and European populations first came into contact in North America. Thus, few genetic markers can be used to categorize an African American's genome into sections with African or European origins because the chromosomal segments of one or the other lineage are long in the admixed population. Therefore, by examining African Americans, it is possible to locate the genomic regions where a high percentage of lineage from either Europeans or Africans is found in MS patients. This suggests that there is an MS variant that varies in frequency between the two ancestral populations. Although this mapping approach was first proposed many years ago, it was not until the development of genetic markers that can distinguish between human populations with varying ancestries that it could be completely put into practice. The susceptibility gene on chromosome 1 should be cloned in future research. It is interesting to note that the normal-appearing white matter (NAWM) revealed a significant elevation of immune-related genes, primarily those involved in signaling and effector activities like lymphocyte activation and disruption of the blood-brain barrier (BBB). These findings confirm the existence of physiological anomalies in NAWM and offer a molecular understanding of the pathogenic mechanisms behind MS. Some researchers investigated the expression of the protein in both silent lesions and acute MS lesions. Genes linked to MHC class II antigen presentation, immunoglobulin production, complement, and pro-inflammatory cytokines were expressed more frequently in both types of lesions. Genes linked to the synthesis of myelin and neurons were underexpressed. Lesions that were silent and active had different expression patterns. It was shown that chronic silent MS lesions had higher levels of α4-integrin; in particular, antibodies to α4-integrin reverse and lower the recurrence rate in experimental autoimmune encephalomyelitis (EAE), and a form of this antibody demonstrated encouraging results when used to treat multiple sclerosis in humans. Chronic silent MS lesions showed increased expression of IgE and IgG Fc receptors. As a result, animals with compromised IgE and IgG Fc receptors experience a less severe EAE than mice of the wild type. According to microarray research, which indicates that Fc receptor transcripts are higher in chronic but not acute MS lesions, these effects became more pronounced on day 20 after the disease was induced.

Only the MS mRNA population exhibited OPN transcripts; control brain mRNA did not. Immunohistochemistry of human MS plaques confirmed the elevated expression of OPN, demonstrating OPN expression in macrophages, microvascular endothelial cells, and the white matter regions surrounding plaques. Mice and rats used as models for relapsing-remitting and monophasic experimental autoimmune encephalomyelitis (EAE), respectively, showed similar expression patterns. OPN-deficient mice were created to examine the significance of OPN in MS. The EAE in these mice was less severe. Using neutralizing antibodies to neutralize OPN also improved EAE, confirming the efficacy of cDNA microarrays in the search for novel MS treatment targets(DiSano et al., 2019). Searches for polymorphisms in the OPN gene linked to MS were prompted by the replication of the increase of OPN levels in MS plaques and in the circulation of MS patients. Polymorphisms in the OPN locus have been linked to elevated circulating OPN levels and the progression of the disease. OPN serves as an illustration of how findings from transcriptomics research could help in the discovery of genetic variations connected to multiple sclerosis. Analysis of the transcriptional profile may also be used to track the course of the disease and the effectiveness of treatment, as well as to investigate the immunological response in multiple sclerosis. However, while using cDNA arrays to analyze the immune response in MS patients, two things should be considered: First, these investigations make the assumption that peripheral changes somehow reflect the condition inside the central nervous system. Second, these investigations are constrained by the typical noise in gene expression, which comes from a variety of sources, including the relative fraction of various blood cell subsets, age, gender, and the time of day the sample was collected.

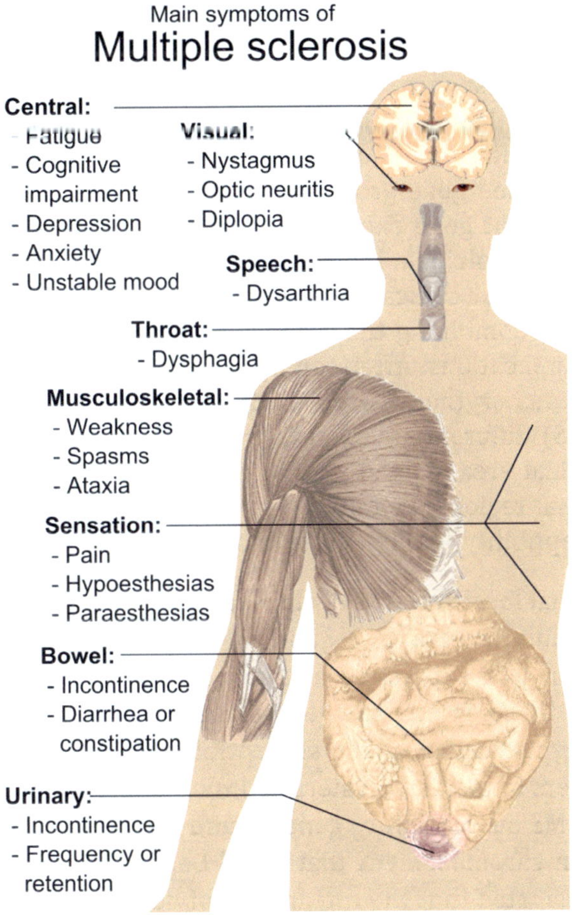

Figure 8.6 Multiple sclerosis

Source: By Mikael Häggström.When using this image in external works, it may be cited as:Häggström, Mikael (2014). "Medical gallery of Mikael Häggström 2014". WikiJournal of Medicine 1 (2). DOI:10.15347/wjm/2014.008. ISSN 2002-4436. Public Domain.orBy Mikael Häggström, used with permission. - All used images are in public domain., Public Domain, https://commons.wikimedia.org/w/index.php?curid=5857315,*Creative Commons License.*

8.11 Gene profiling

The gene expression profiling can be utilized to categorize patients based on various clinical parameters, such as therapeutic responders or non-responders. Although interferon (IFN) is frequently used to treat multiple sclerosis (MS) (Figure 8.6), neither its exact mode of action nor the biomarkers that would enable the identification of people who would benefit from it are known. The effects of IFN therapy on the transcriptional activity of monocyte-depleted PBMC were investigated using cDNA microarrays. According to this investigation, there are prominent alterations in the expression of genes related to the antiviral response, IFN signaling, and indicators of lymphocyte activation after one hour of IFN treatment. These investigations gave a molecular basis of how IFN affected individuals with RRMS, and they were further expanded to find transcriptional markers linked to a positive response to IFN treatment. They showed that certain patterns of gene expression are present in MS patients who respond well to IFN treatment, as determined by clinical disease activity and MRI scans. To identify MS patients who are likely to respond to IFN treatment, researchers identified gene groups whose expression has a predictive value based on these data. Research shows that gene expression profiling can be utilized to choose a treatment plan that fits the patient's metabolism in the treatment of multiple sclerosis. Research studies made use of an approach (RT-PCR) that clinical labs could use, making it easier to apply the findings to routine medical procedures. Combining the data from genomes and transcriptomics research can yield novel theories and applications. After comparing the genes that lymphocytes in rheumatoid arthritis (RA), systemic lupus erythematosus (SLE), insulin-dependent diabetic mellitus (IDDM), and multiple sclerosis (MS) differentially expressed, researchers concluded that these genes are grouped inside chromosomal areas in the genome. They discovered that genetic linkage studies could map the chromosomal regions containing the genes differentially expressed in autoimmune disorders to disease susceptibility loci linked to those diseases.

These findings imply that local patterns of chromatin condensation or shared genetic regulatory elements may be responsible for the co-regulation of disease-associated gene expression. The genetic association between gene expression and genetic linkage in multiple sclerosis was recently investigated. They started by compiling the gene expression data that was available for both MS and EAE, then overlapping it with all of the susceptibility loci that were known to exist in both conditions. Some researchers found that clusters of differentially expressed genes in MS and murine EAE overlapped with the MS susceptibility genes found in the MHC locus(Mix et al., 2004). They also discovered an area on chromosome X that could be involved in the sexual dimorphism seen in MS. Therefore, it is anticipated that the integration of data produced by several platforms, such as transcriptomics, genomes, and proteomics, will enhance our comprehension of the mechanisms underlying MS. To activate peptide-specific T cells and track cytokine secretion or adhesion, MHC arrays were recently developed based on the immobilization of peptide/MHC tetramers. The high frequency of polymorphisms on the MHC locus limits their use in the study of human immunology. However, scientists have recently employed these arrays to describe the cellular response in humans who have received a tumor treatment. Antibodies specific to phosphorylated or dephosphorylated proteins involved in signaling transduction pathways of interest are used to probe arrays of spotted lysates made from primary cells, which make up reverse phase arrays. It is possible to create comprehensive signaling maps that describe the molecular processes that result in the activation of a particular cell population by combining various antibodies and inhibitors of particular signal transduction pathways. Recently, CD4 CD25 regulatory T cells (Treg) have been studied using this methodology. These arrays may help identify signaling abnormalities in MS patient immune systems and how these pathways are altered in immuno-modulatory regimes, as Treg function defects have been reported in MS patients.

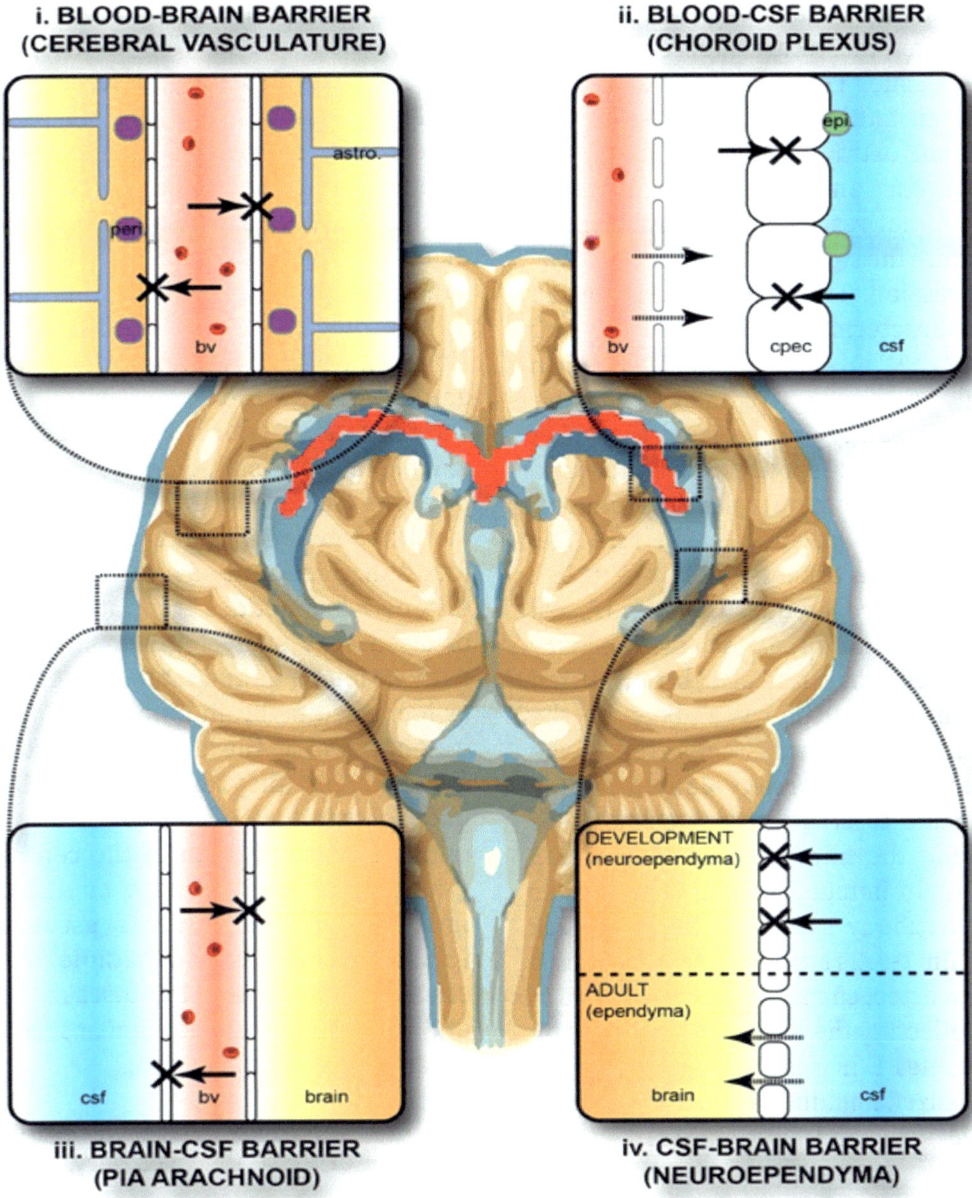

Figure 8.7 Blood-brain barrier

Source: https://upload.wikimedia.org/wikipedia/commons/b/b5/Protective_barriers_of_the_brain.jpg,*Creative Commons License.*

8.12 Blood-brain barrier and other aspects

Autoimmune T-cells must express surface molecules that enable them to penetrate the blood-brain barrier (Figure 8.7) and start an infection to enter the central nervous system and destroy tissue. The beneficial effects of natalizumab, an antibody to α4 integrin that prevents T cell extravasation to the central nervous system and has demonstrated encouraging initial results in the treatment of MS, demonstrate the significance of this pathway for MS progression. Therefore, describing the adhesion characteristics displayed by the various cell types in MS patients may aid in anticipating and tracking treatment response as well as anticipating and averting the onset of relapses. Antibody responses are believed to reflect the activity of the T cell compartment, which makes them of interest in MS. The antibodies may have a pathogenic role in MS. These antibodies are produced by intrathecal germinal centers that appear to form tertiary lymph nodes, but they can also be produced by B cells in the periphery and go to the infected central nervous system through the damaged blood-brain barrier. Many attempts have been made to create novel technologies for monitoring the humoral response in MS patients and autoimmunity since it is simpler to evaluate antibody reactivity than to track antigen-specific T-cell responses. Antigen arrays can be used to detect changes in the repertoire of antibodies reflecting the antigen dissemination that accompanies EAE progression(Kidd et al., 2008). Customized immunomodulatory vaccines were created using the data gathered on the level of antigen spreading observed in each animal to suppress EAE. As demonstrated for other autoimmune disorders like RA, autoimmune diabetes, and SLE, future research should examine the antibody response in the serum of MS patients, looking for patterns of antibody reactivity that predict the progression of MS or the response to therapy. Antigen arrays may also be employed to examine the antibody repertoire to identify novel targets for immunomodulation and, consequently, novel targets of the MS autoimmune attack. Antigen arrays may be utilized to detect antibody patterns associated with the various types of multiple sclerosis as well as the pathology at the lesion site. Proteomic research has revealed novel processes underlying MS pathogenesis. Researchers discovered distinct autoantibody patterns that set Relapsing-Remitting MS (RRMS); Secondary-Progressive MS (SPMS); Primary-Progressive MS (PPMS) apart from healthy controls as well as other autoimmune or neurological-driven conditions like lupus erythematosus, Alzheimer's disease, and adrenoleukodystrophy. Autoantibodies and heat shock proteins, which were absent from PPMS and SPMS, were characteristic of RRMS. Distinct patterns of response to CNS antigens were identified in RRMS, SPMS, and PPMS. Scientists found distinct antibody patterns to lipids and CNS-derived peptides associated with each type of disease by analyzing sera from individuals with various immunopathologic patterns of MS as identified by brain biopsy. A more thorough examination of these lipids' function in EAE revealed that they directly contribute to the pathophysiology of MS by stimulating the innate immune system of the central nervous system. The identification of distinct serum immunological signatures associated with various MS stages and pathologic processes offers a way to track the disease, describe its immunopathogenic mechanisms, and identify potential treatment targets.

The individual clinical presentation and outcome of these diseases vary, most likely as a result of variations in genetic susceptibility, environmental factor exposure, intestinal commensal bacteria, and the intestinal immune system. While there are some similarities between CD and UC, there are also significant variances, and it is still unclear whether the two conditions are molecularly linked enough to be grouped together as irritable bowel disease (IBD). Nevertheless, there is evidence that the chronic intestinal inflammation is caused by a dysregulated mucosal immune response, which may have been brought on by a malfunctioning (immunological) intestinal barrier. Several factors influence the chance of developing IBD. Several unrelated environmental factors, such as smoking, oral contraception, diet, breastfeeding, drugs, stress, microbial agents, intestinal permeability, and appendectomy, have been linked to IBD in addition to genetic factors. However, the only environmental risk factor for IBD that has been proven is smoking, which lowers the risk of UC while raising the risk of CD. There is a significant genetic component to IBD, but it appears to be more visible in CD than in UC. A combination of distinct clinical, endoscopic, and pathological findings can be used to identify CD. In CD patients, radiographic examinations serve as a supplement to endoscopic findings.

REFERENCES

1. Åkerblom, H. K., Virtanen, S. M., Ilonen, J., Savilahti, E., Vaarala, O., Reunanen, A., Teramo, K., Hämäläinen, A.-M., Paronen, J., Riikjärv, M.-A., Ormisson, A., Ludvigsson, J., Dosch, H.-M., Hakulinen, T., Knip, M., & National TRIGR Study Groups. (2005). Dietary manipulation of beta cell autoimmunity in infants at increased risk of type 1 diabetes: A pilot study. *Diabetologia*, *48*(5), 829–837. https://doi.org/10.1007/s00125-005-1733-3

2. Al-Anazi, M. R., Matou-Nasri, S., Abdo, A. A., Sanai, F. M., Khan, M. Q., Albenmousa, A., Al-Ashgar, H. I., Khalaf, N. Z., Al-Ahdal, M. N., & Al-Qahtani, A. A. (2014). Variations in DEPDC5 gene and its association with chronic hepatitis C virus infection in Saudi Arabia. *BMC Infectious Diseases*, *14*(1), 632. https://doi.org/10.1186/s12879-014-0632-y

3. Altmeier, S., & LeibundGut-Landmann, S. (2017). Immunity to Fungal Infections. In A. Carvalho (Ed.), *Immunogenetics of Fungal Diseases* (pp. 35–83). Springer International Publishing. https://doi.org/10.1007/978-3-319-50842-9_2

4. Ambegaokar, S. S., Roy, B., & Jackson, G. R. (2010). Neurodegenerative models in *Drosophila:* Polyglutamine disorders, Parkinson disease, and amyotrophic lateral sclerosis. *Neurobiology of Disease*, *40*(1), 29–39. https://doi.org/10.1016/j.nbd.2010.05.026

5. Aringer, M. (2020). Inflammatory markers in systemic lupus erythematosus. *Journal of Autoimmunity*, *110*, 102374. https://doi.org/10.1016/j.jaut.2019.102374

6. Averbeck, M., Gebhardt, C., Emmrich, F., Treudler, R., & Simon, J. C. (2007). Immunologic Principles of Allergic Disease. *JDDG: Journal Der Deutschen Dermatologischen Gesellschaft*, *5*(11), 1015–1027. https://doi.org/10.1111/j.1610-0387.2007.06538.x

7. Ayala-Fontánez, N., Soler, D. C., & McCormick, T. S. (2016). Current knowledge on psoriasis and autoimmune diseases. *Psoriasis: Targets and Therapy*, *6*, 7–32. https://doi.org/10.2147/PTT.S64950

8. Balhara, J., & Gounni, A. S. (2012). The alveolar macrophages in asthma: A double-edged sword. *Mucosal Immunology*, *5*(6), 605–609. https://doi.org/10.1038/mi.2012.74

9. Basak, S., & Hoffmann, A. (2008). Crosstalk via the NF-κB signaling system. *Cytokine & Growth Factor Reviews*, *19*(3), 187–197. https://doi.org/10.1016/j.cytogfr.2008.04.005

10. Bentley, G. A., & Mariuzza, R. A. (1996). THE STRUCTURE OF THE T CELL ANTIGEN RECEPTOR. *Annual Review of Immunology*, *14*(Volume 14, 1996), 563–590. https://doi.org/10.1146/annurev.immunol.14.1.563

11. Berezin, V., Walmod, P. S., Filippov, M., & Dityatev, A. (2014). Chapter 15—Targeting of ECM molecules and their metabolizing enzymes and receptors for the treatment of CNS diseases. In A. Dityatev, B. Wehrle-Haller, & A. Pitkänen (Eds.), *Progress in Brain Research* (Vol. 214, pp. 353–388). Elsevier. https://doi.org/10.1016/B978-0-444-63486-3.00015-3

12. Bonita, R. E., Rose, N. R., Rasooly, L., Caturegli, P., & Burek, C. L. (2002). Adhesion Molecules as Susceptibility Factors in Spontaneous Autoimmune Thyroiditis in the NOD-H2h4 Mouse. *Experimental and Molecular Pathology*, *73*(3), 155–163. https://doi.org/10.1006/exmp.2002.2470

13. Boyman, O., Krieg, C., Homann, D., & Sprent, J. (2012). Homeostatic maintenance of T cells and natural killer cells. *Cellular and Molecular Life Sciences*, *69*(10), 1597–1608. https://doi.org/10.1007/s00018-012-0968-7

14. Brix, T. H., Hansen, P. S., Hegedüs, L., & Wenzel, B. E. (2008). Too early to dismiss *Yersinia enterocolitica* infection in the aetiology of Graves' disease: Evidence from a twin case–control study. *Clinical Endocrinology*, *69*(3), 491–496. https://doi.org/10.1111/j.1365-2265.2008.03227.x

15. Burek, C. L., & Rose, N. R. (2008). Autoimmune thyroiditis and ROS. *Autoimmunity Reviews*, *7*(7), 530–537. https://doi.org/10.1016/j.autrev.2008.04.006

16. Buse, E., & Markert, U. R. (2019). The immunology of the macaque placenta: A detailed analysis and critical comparison with the human placenta. *Critical Reviews in Clinical Laboratory Sciences*, *56*(2), 118–145. https://doi.org/10.1080/10408363.2018.1538200

17. Castley, A. S. L., & Martinez, O. P. (2012). Molecular Analysis of Complement Component C4 Gene Copy Number. In F. T. Christiansen & B. D. Tait (Eds.), *Immunogenetics: Methods and Applications in Clinical Practice* (pp. 159–171). Humana Press. https://doi.org/10.1007/978-1-61779-842-9_9

18. Chang, H. Y., & Yang, X. (2000). Proteases for Cell Suicide: Functions and Regulation of Caspases. *Microbiology and Molecular Biology Reviews*, *64*(4), 821–846. https://doi.org/10.1128/mmbr.64.4.821-846.2000

19. Chauhan, S. K., Rai, R., Singh, V. V., Rai, M., & Rai, G. (2015). Differential clearance mechanisms, neutrophil extracellular trap degradation and phagocytosis, are operative in systemic lupus erythematosus patients with distinct autoantibody specificities. *Immunology Letters*, *168*(2), 254–259. https://doi.org/10.1016/j.imlet.2015.09.016

20. Chen, T., & Gao, C. (2024). Innate immune signal transduction pathways to fungal infection: Components and regulation. *Cell Insight*, *3*(3), 100154. https://doi.org/10.1016/j.cellin.2024.100154

21. Chen, Z. J. (2012). Ubiquitination in signaling to and activation of IKK. *Immunological Reviews*, *246*(1), 95–106. https://doi.org/10.1111/j.1600-065X.2012.01108.x

22. Childers, D. S., Avelar, G. M., Bain, J. M., Larcombe, D. E., Pradhan, A., Budge, S., Heaney, H., & Brown, A. J. P. (2020). Impact of the Environment upon the *Candida albicans* Cell Wall and Resultant Effects upon Immune Surveillance. In J.-P. Latgé (Ed.), *The Fungal Cell Wall: An Armour and a Weapon for Human Fungal Pathogens* (pp. 297–330). Springer International Publishing. https://doi.org/10.1007/82_2019_182

23. Chou, K.-C., Tomasselli, A. G., & Heinrikson, R. L. (2000). Prediction of the tertiary structure of a caspase-9/inhibitor complex. *FEBS Letters*, *470*(3), 249–256. https://doi.org/10.1016/S0014-5793(00)01333-8

24. Christian, F., Smith, E. L., & Carmody, R. J. (2016). The Regulation of NF-κB Subunits by Phosphorylation. *Cells*, *5*(1), Article 1. https://doi.org/10.3390/cells5010012

25. Ciarimboli, G. (2016). Introduction to the Cellular Transport of Organic Cations. In G. Ciarimboli, S. Gautron, & E. Schlatter (Eds.), *Organic Cation Transporters: Integration of Physiology, Pathology, and Pharmacology* (pp. 1–47). Springer International Publishing. https://doi.org/10.1007/978-3-319-23793-0_1

26. Conigliaro, P., Chimenti, M. S., Triggianese, P., Sunzini, F., Novelli, L., Perricone, C., & Perricone, R. (2016). Autoantibodies in inflammatory arthritis. *Autoimmunity Reviews*, *15*(7), 673–683. https://doi.org/10.1016/j.autrev.2016.03.003

27. Copley, M. S., Waldron, M., Athans, V., Welch, S. C., Brizendine, K. D., Cober, E., & Siebenaller, C. (2020). Itraconazole vs. posaconazole for antifungal prophylaxis in patients with acute myeloid leukemia undergoing intensive chemotherapy: A retrospective study. *International Journal of Antimicrobial Agents*, *55*(3), 105886. https://doi.org/10.1016/j.ijantimicag.2020.105886

28. Courtois, G., & Fauvarque, M.-O. (2018). The Many Roles of Ubiquitin in NF-κB Signaling. *Biomedicines*, *6*(2), Article 2. https://doi.org/10.3390/biomedicines6020043

29. Crespo, Â. C., van der Zwan, A., Ramalho-Santos, J., Strominger, J. L., & Tilburgs, T. (2017). Cytotoxic potential of decidual NK cells and CD8+ T cells awakened by infections. *Journal of Reproductive Immunology*, *119*, 85–90. https://doi.org/10.1016/j.jri.2016.08.001

30. Cyna, W., Wojciechowska, A., Szybiak-Skora, W., & Lacka, K. (2024). The Impact of Environmental Factors on the Development of Autoimmune Thyroiditis—Review. *Biomedicines*, *12*(8), Article 8. https://doi.org/10.3390/biomedicines12081788

31. de Almeida, B. S., Muniz, Y. C. N., Prompt, A. H., Castelli, E. C., Mendes-Junior, C. T., & Donadi, E. A. (2018). Genetic association between *HLA-G* 14-bp polymorphism and diseases: A systematic review and meta-analysis. *Human Immunology*, *79*(10), 724–735. https://doi.org/10.1016/j.humimm.2018.08.003

32. de Repentigny, L., Lewandowski, D., & Jolicoeur, P. (2004). Immunopathogenesis of Oropharyngeal Candidiasis in Human Immunodeficiency Virus Infection. *Clinical Microbiology Reviews*, *17*(4), 729–759. https://doi.org/10.1128/cmr.17.4.729-759.2004

33. Delacher, M., Schreiber, L., Richards, D. M., Farah, C., Feuerer, M., & Huehn, J. (2014). Transcriptional Control of Regulatory T cells. In W. Ellmeier & I. Taniuchi (Eds.), *Transcriptional Control of Lineage Differentiation in Immune Cells* (pp. 83–124). Springer International Publishing. https://doi.org/10.1007/82_2014_373

34. Devendra, D., & Eisenbarth, G. S. (2004). Interferon alpha—A potential link in the pathogenesis of viral-induced type 1 diabetes and autoimmunity. *Clinical Immunology*, *111*(3), 225–233. https://doi.org/10.1016/j.clim.2004.01.008

35. DiSano, K. D., Linzey, M. R., Royce, D. B., Pachner, A. R., & Gilli, F. (2019). Differential neuro-immune patterns in two clinically relevant murine models of multiple sclerosis. *Journal of Neuroinflammation*, *16*(1), 109. https://doi.org/10.1186/s12974-019-1501-9

36. Donath, M. Y., Størling, J., Maedler, K., & Mandrup-Poulsen, T. (2003). Inflammatory mediators and islet β-cell failure: A link between type 1 and type 2 diabetes. *Journal of Molecular Medicine, 81*(8), 455–470. https://doi.org/10.1007/s00109-003-0450-y
37. Dunckley, H. (2012). HLA Typing by SSO and SSP Methods. In F. T. Christiansen & B. D. Tait (Eds.), *Immunogenetics: Methods and Applications in Clinical Practice* (pp. 9–25). Humana Press. https://doi.org/10.1007/978-1-61779-842-9_2
38. Duré, M., & Macian, F. (2009). IL-2 signaling prevents T cell anergy by inhibiting the expression of anergy-inducing genes. *Molecular Immunology, 46*(5), 999–1006. https://doi.org/10.1016/j.molimm.2008.09.029
39. Dzopalic, T., Rajkovic, I., Dragicevic, A., & Colic, M. (2012). The response of human dendritic cells to co-ligation of pattern-recognition receptors. *Immunologic Research, 52*(1), 20–33. https://doi.org/10.1007/s12026-012-8279-5
40. Ebert, P. J. R., Li, Q.-J., Huppa, J. B., & Davis, M. M. (2010). Functional Development of the T Cell Receptor for Antigen. In A. Liston (Ed.), *Progress in Molecular Biology and Translational Science* (Vol. 92, pp. 65–100). Academic Press. https://doi.org/10.1016/S1877-1173(10)92004-8
41. Edwards, K. M., Davis, J. E., Browne, K. A., Sutton, V. R., & Trapani, J. A. (1999). Anti-viral strategies of cytotoxic T lymphocytes are manifested through a variety of granule-bound pathways of apoptosis induction. *Immunology & Cell Biology, 77*(1), 76–89. https://doi.org/10.1046/j.1440-1711.1999.00799.x
42. El-Benhawy, S. A., Fahmy, E. I., Mahdy, S. M., Khedr, G. H., Sarhan, A. S., Nafady, M. H., Yousef Selim, Y. A., Salem, T. M., Abu-Samra, N., & El Khadry, H. A. (2022). Assessment of thyroid gland hormones and ultrasonographic abnormalities in medical staff occupationally exposed to ionizing radiation. *BMC Endocrine Disorders, 22*(1), 287. https://doi.org/10.1186/s12902-022-01196-z
43. Enoch, D. A., Yang, H., Aliyu, S. H., & Micallef, C. (2017). The Changing Epidemiology of Invasive Fungal Infections. In T. Lion (Ed.), *Human Fungal Pathogen Identification: Methods and Protocols* (pp. 17–65). Springer. https://doi.org/10.1007/978-1-4939-6515-1_2
44. Erlich, H. (2012). HLA DNA typing: Past, present, and future. *Tissue Antigens, 80*(1), 1–11. https://doi.org/10.1111/j.1399-0039.2012.01881.x
45. Eskes, S. A., & Wiersinga, W. M. (2009). Amiodarone and thyroid. *Best Practice & Research Clinical Endocrinology & Metabolism, 23*(6), 735–751. https://doi.org/10.1016/j.beem.2009.07.001
46. Eun, A. J.-C., Seoh, M.-L., & Wong, S.-M. (2000). Simultaneous quantitation of two orchid viruses by the TaqMan® real-time RT-PCR. *Journal of Virological Methods, 87*(1), 151–160. https://doi.org/10.1016/S0166-0934(00)00161-0
47. Fagerlund, R., Melén, K., Cao, X., & Julkunen, I. (2008). NF-κB p52, RelB and c-Rel are transported into the nucleus via a subset of importin α molecules. *Cellular Signalling, 20*(8), 1442–1451. https://doi.org/10.1016/j.cellsig.2008.03.012
48. Fan, Y., He, H., Dong, Y., & Pan, H. (2013). Hyphae-Specific Genes HGC1, ALS3, HWP1, and ECE1 and Relevant Signaling Pathways in Candida albicans. *Mycopathologia, 176*(5), 329–335. https://doi.org/10.1007/s11046-013-9684-6
49. Fink, P. J., & Bevan, M. J. (1995). Positive Selection of Thymocytes. In F. J. Dixon (Ed.), *Advances in Immunology* (Vol. 59, pp. 99–134). Academic Press. https://doi.org/10.1016/S0065-2776(08)60630-6

50. Fischer, B., Coelho, D., Dufour, P., Bergerat, J.-P., Denis, J.-M., Gueulette, J., & Bischoff, P. (2003). Caspase 8-mediated cleavage of the pro-apoptotic BCL-2 family member BID in p53-dependent apoptosis. *Biochemical and Biophysical Research Communications*, *306*(2), 516–522. https://doi.org/10.1016/S0006-291X(03)01004-0

51. Frandji, P., Tkaczyk, C., Oskeritzian, C., David, B., Desaymard, C., & Mécheri, S. (1996). Exogenous and endogenous antigens are differentially presented by mast cells to CD4+ T lymphocytes. *European Journal of Immunology*, *26*(10), 2517–2528. https://doi.org/10.1002/eji.1830261036

52. Fürnrohr, B. G., Sheriff, A., Munoz, L., von Briesen, H., Urbonaviciute, V., Neubert, K., Kalden, J. R., Herrmann, M., & Voll, R. E. (2005). Signals, receptors, and cytokines involved in the immunomodulatory and anti-inflammatory properties of apoptotic cells. *Signal Transduction*, *5*(6), 356–365. https://doi.org/10.1002/sita.200500071

53. Gaastra, W., & Oudega, B. (1983). The Determination of DNA Sequences. In J. M. Walker & W. Gaastra (Eds.), *Techniques in Molecular Biology* (pp. 287–307). Springer Netherlands. https://doi.org/10.1007/978-94-011-6563-1_16

54. Gea-Banacloche, J. (2017). Granulocyte transfusions: A concise review for practitioners. *Cytotherapy*, *19*(11), 1256–1269. https://doi.org/10.1016/j.jcyt.2017.08.012

55. Geraghty, D. E., Daza, R., Williams, L. M., Vu, Q., & Ishitani, A. (2002). Genetics of the immune response: Identifying immune variation within the MHC and throughout the genome. *Immunological Reviews*, *190*(1), 69–85. https://doi.org/10.1034/j.1600-065X.2002.19006.x

56. Geraghty, L., Figtree, G. A., Schutte, A. E., Patel, S., Woodward, M., & Arnott, C. (2021). Cardiovascular Disease in Women: From Pathophysiology to Novel and Emerging Risk Factors. *Heart, Lung and Circulation*, *30*(1), 9–17. https://doi.org/10.1016/j.hlc.2020.05.108

57. Gnat, S., Łagowski, D., & Nowakiewicz, A. (2021). Genetic Predisposition and its Heredity in the Context of Increased Prevalence of Dermatophytoses. *Mycopathologia*, *186*(2), 163–176. https://doi.org/10.1007/s11046-021-00529-1

58. Gow, N. A. R., Latge, J.-P., & Munro, C. A. (2017). The Fungal Cell Wall: Structure, Biosynthesis, and Function. *Microbiology Spectrum*, *5*(3), 10.1128/microbiolspec.funk-0035–2016. https://doi.org/10.1128/microbiolspec.funk-0035-2016

59. Gupta, P. K. (2004). Pesticide exposure—Indian scene. *Toxicology*, *198*(1), 83–90. https://doi.org/10.1016/j.tox.2004.01.021

60. Gupta, R. K., & Gupta, G. S. (2012). Mannose Receptor Family: R-Type Lectins. In G. S. Gupta (Ed.), *Animal Lectins: Form, Function and Clinical Applications* (pp. 331–347). Springer. https://doi.org/10.1007/978-3-7091-1065-2_15

61. Haks, M. C., Oosterwegel, M. A., Blom, B., Spits, H. M., & Kruisbeek, A. M. (1999). Cell-fate decisions in early T cell development: Regulation by cytokine receptors and the pre-TCR. *Seminars in Immunology*, *11*(1), 23–37. https://doi.org/10.1006/smim.1998.0153

62. Hart, P. A., Zen, Y., & Chari, S. T. (2015). Recent Advances in Autoimmune Pancreatitis. *Gastroenterology*, *149*(1), 39–51. https://doi.org/10.1053/j.gastro.2015.03.010

63. Hassan, MD. I., & Ahmad, F. (2011). Chapter 6—Structural diversity of class I MHC-like molecules and its implications in binding specificities. In R. Donev (Ed.), *Advances in Protein Chemistry and Structural Biology* (Vol. 83, pp. 223–270). Academic Press. https://doi.org/10.1016/B978-0-12-381262-9.00006-9

64. Hermann, E., Meyer zum Büschenfelde, K.-H., Fleischer, B., & Yu, D. T. Y. (1993). HLA-B27-restricted CD8 T cells derived from synovial fluids of patients with reactive arthritis and ankylosing spondylitis. *The Lancet, 342*(8872), 646–650. https://doi.org/10.1016/0140-6736(93)91760-J

65. Héron, E., Deloukas, P., & van Loon, A. P. G. M. (1995). The Complete Exon-Intron Structure of the 156-kb Human Gene *NFKB1*, Which Encodes the p105 and p50 Proteins of Transcription Factors NF-κB and IκB-γ: Implications for NF-κB-Mediated Signal Transduction. *Genomics, 30*(3), 493–505. https://doi.org/10.1006/geno.1995.1270

66. Hohenester, E., & Engel, J. (2002). Domain structure and organisation in extracellular matrix proteins. *Matrix Biology, 21*(2), 115–128. https://doi.org/10.1016/S0945-053X(01)00191-3

67. Hollenbach, J. A., Mack, S. J., Thomson, G., & Gourraud, P.-A. (2012). Analytical Methods for Disease Association Studies with Immunogenetic Data. In F. T. Christiansen & B. D. Tait (Eds.), *Immunogenetics: Methods and Applications in Clinical Practice* (pp. 245–266). Humana Press. https://doi.org/10.1007/978-1-61779-842-9_14

68. Honkanen, H., Oikarinen, S., Nurminen, N., Laitinen, O. H., Huhtala, H., Lehtonen, J., Ruokoranta, T., Hankaniemi, M. M., Lecouturier, V., Almond, J. W., Tauriainen, S., Simell, O., Ilonen, J., Veijola, R., Viskari, H., Knip, M., & Hyöty, H. (2017). Detection of enteroviruses in stools precedes islet autoimmunity by several months: Possible evidence for slowly operating mechanisms in virus-induced autoimmunity. *Diabetologia, 60*(3), 424–431. https://doi.org/10.1007/s00125-016-4177-z

69. Horowitz, L. B., & Shaham, S. (2024). *Apoptotic and Nonapoptotic Cell Death in Caenorhabditis elegans Development.* https://doi.org/10.1146/annurev-genet-111523-102051

70. Huehn, J., & Beyer, M. (2015). Epigenetic and transcriptional control of Foxp3+ regulatory T cells. *Seminars in Immunology, 27*(1), 10–18. https://doi.org/10.1016/j.smim.2015.02.002

71. Irwin, M. R. (1976). The beginnings of immunogenetics. *Immunogenetics, 3*(1), 1–13. https://doi.org/10.1007/BF01576934

72. Javidan, M., Amiri, A. M., Koohi, N., Joudaki, N., Bashirrohelleh, M. A., Pirsadeghi, A., Biregani, A. F., Rashno, M., Dehcheshmeh, M. G., Sharifat, M., Khodadadi, A., & Mafakher, L. (2024). Restoring immune balance with Tregitopes: A new approach to treating immunological disorders. *Biomedicine & Pharmacotherapy, 177*, 116983. https://doi.org/10.1016/j.biopha.2024.116983

73. Jiang, H., & Chess, L. (2000). The Specific Regulation Of Immune Responses By CD8+ T Cells Restricted By The MHC Class Ib Molecule, Qa-1. *Annual Review of Immunology, 18*(Volume 18, 2000), 185–216. https://doi.org/10.1146/annurev.immunol.18.1.185

74. Jorgovanovic, D., Song, M., Wang, L., & Zhang, Y. (2020). Roles of IFN-γ in tumor progression and regression: A review. *Biomarker Research, 8*(1), 49. https://doi.org/10.1186/s40364-020-00228-x

75. Kashem, S. W., Haniffa, M., & Kaplan, D. H. (2017). Antigen-Presenting Cells in the Skin. *Annual Review of Immunology, 35*(Volume 35, 2017), 469–499. https://doi.org/10.1146/annurev-immunol-051116-052215

76. Keresztes, A., & Streicher, J. M. (2017). Synergistic interaction of the cannabinoid and death receptor systems – a potential target for future cancer therapies? *FEBS Letters, 591*(20), 3235–3251. https://doi.org/10.1002/1873-3468.12863

77. Kesavardhana, S., Malireddi, R. K. S., & Kanneganti, T.-D. (2020). Caspases in Cell Death, Inflammation, and Pyroptosis. *Annual Review of Immunology*, *38*(Volume 38, 2020), 567–595. https://doi.org/10.1146/annurev-immunol-073119-095439

78. Kidd, B. A., Ho, P. P., Sharpe, O., Zhao, X., Tomooka, B. H., Kanter, J. L., Steinman, L., & Robinson, W. H. (2008). Epitope spreading to citrullinated antigens in mouse models of autoimmune arthritis and demyelination. *Arthritis Research & Therapy*, *10*(5), R119. https://doi.org/10.1186/ar2523

79. Knip, M., Luopajärvi, K., & Härkönen, T. (2017). Early life origin of type 1 diabetes. *Seminars in Immunopathology*, *39*(6), 653–667. https://doi.org/10.1007/s00281-017-0665-6

80. Knip, M., & Siljander, H. (2008). Autoimmune mechanisms in type 1 diabetes. *Autoimmunity Reviews*, *7*(7), 550–557. https://doi.org/10.1016/j.autrev.2008.04.008

81. Koriem, K. M. M. (2016). Multiple sclerosis: New insights and trends. *Asian Pacific Journal of Tropical Biomedicine*, *6*(5), 429–440. https://doi.org/10.1016/j.apjtb.2016.03.009

82. Kotenko, S. V. (2011). IFN-λs. *Current Opinion in Immunology*, *23*(5), 583–590. https://doi.org/10.1016/j.coi.2011.07.007

83. Lakhani, S., Lu, B., & Flavell, R. A. (2002). Caspase Knockouts: Matters of Life and Death. In *Apoptosis and Autoimmunity* (pp. 13–35). John Wiley & Sons, Ltd. https://doi.org/10.1002/3527601457.ch2

84. Lee, H.-M., Bautista, J. L., & Hsieh, C.-S. (2011). Chapter 2—Thymic and Peripheral Differentiation of Regulatory T Cells. In R. Alexander & S. Shimon (Eds.), *Advances in Immunology* (Vol. 112, pp. 25–71). Academic Press. https://doi.org/10.1016/B978-0-12-387827-4.00002-4

85. Lee, Y. K., Mukasa, R., Hatton, R. D., & Weaver, C. T. (2009). Developmental plasticity of Th17 and Treg cells. *Current Opinion in Immunology*, *21*(3), 274–280. https://doi.org/10.1016/j.coi.2009.05.021

86. Lehman, H. K., & Segal, B. H. (2020). The role of neutrophils in host defense and disease. *Journal of Allergy and Clinical Immunology*, *145*(6), 1535–1544. https://doi.org/10.1016/j.jaci.2020.02.038

87. Lemoine, S., Morva, A., Youinou, P., & Jamin, C. (2011). Human T cells induce their own regulation through activation of B cells. *Journal of Autoimmunity*, *36*(3), 228–238. https://doi.org/10.1016/j.jaut.2011.01.005

88. Li, M. O., Wan, Y. Y., Sanjabi, S., Robertson, A.-K. L., & Flavell, R. A. (2006). TRANSFORMING GROWTH FACTOR-β REGULATION OF IMMUNE RESPONSES. *Annual Review of Immunology*, *24*(Volume 24, 2006), 99–146. https://doi.org/10.1146/annurev.immunol.24.021605.090737

89. Li, W. Q., Guszczynski, T., Hixon, J. A., & Durum, S. K. (2010). Interleukin-7 Regulates Bim Proapoptotic Activity in Peripheral T-Cell Survival. *Molecular and Cellular Biology*, *30*(3), 590–600. https://doi.org/10.1128/MCB.01006-09

90. Lin, P. L., & Flynn, J. L. (2015). CD8 T cells and *Mycobacterium tuberculosis* infection. *Seminars in Immunopathology*, *37*(3), 239–249. https://doi.org/10.1007/s00281-015-0490-8

91. Lin, Y., Ren, L., Wang, W., Di, J., Zeng, S., & Saito, S. (2009). Effect of TLR3 and TLR7 activation in uterine NK cells from non-obese diabetic (NOD) mice. *Journal of Reproductive Immunology*, *82*(1), 12–23. https://doi.org/10.1016/j.jri.2009.03.004

92. Liu, Q. A., & Hengartner, M. O. (1999). The Molecular Mechanism of Programmed Cell Death in C. elegans. *Annals of the New York Academy of Sciences, 887*(1), 92–104. https://doi.org/10.1111/j.1749-6632.1999.tb07925.x

93. Lleo, A., Marzorati, S., Anaya, J.-M., & Gershwin, M. E. (2017). Primary biliary cholangitis: A comprehensive overview. *Hepatology International, 11*(6), 485–499. https://doi.org/10.1007/s12072-017-9830-1

94. Lockhart, S. R., Toda, M., Benedict, K., Caceres, D. H., & Litvintseva, A. P. (2021). Endemic and Other Dimorphic Mycoses in The Americas. *Journal of Fungi, 7*(2), Article 2. https://doi.org/10.3390/jof7020151

95. Loh, J. T., & Lam, K.-P. (2023). Fungal infections: Immune defense, immunotherapies and vaccines. *Advanced Drug Delivery Reviews, 196*, 114775. https://doi.org/10.1016/j.addr.2023.114775

96. Long, H., Yin, H., Wang, L., Gershwin, M. E., & Lu, Q. (2016). The critical role of epigenetics in systemic lupus erythematosus and autoimmunity. *Journal of Autoimmunity, 74*, 118–138. https://doi.org/10.1016/j.jaut.2016.06.020

97. Ma, Q., Pradhan, A., Leaves, I., Hickey, E., Roselletti, E., Dambuza, I., Larcombe, D. E., de Assis, L. J., Wilson, D., Erwig, L. P., Netea, M. G., Childers, D. S., Brown, G. D., Gow, N. A. R., & Brown, A. J. P. (2024). Impact of secreted glucanases upon the cell surface and fitness of *Candida albicans* during colonisation and infection. *The Cell Surface, 11*, 100128. https://doi.org/10.1016/j.tcsw.2024.100128

98. Mahnke, K., Bedke, T., & Enk, A. H. (2007). Regulatory conversation between antigen presenting cells and regulatory T cells enhance immune suppression. *Cellular Immunology, 250*(1), 1–13. https://doi.org/10.1016/j.cellimm.2008.01.004

99. Masuda, E. S., Imamura, R., Amasaki, Y., Arai, K., & Arai, N. (1998). Signalling into the T-Cell Nucleus: NFAT Regulation. *Cellular Signalling, 10*(9), 599–611. https://doi.org/10.1016/S0898-6568(98)00019-9

100. McCarthy, N., Mercer, J., & Bennett, M. (2001). APOPTOTIC PROTEINS: P53 and c-myc Related Pathways. *Cardiology Clinics, 19*(1), 75–89. https://doi.org/10.1016/S0733-8651(05)70196-X

101. McHugh, M. D., Park, J., Uhrich, R., Gao, W., Horwitz, D. A., & Fahmy, T. M. (2015). Paracrine co-delivery of TGF-β and IL-2 using CD4-targeted nanoparticles for induction and maintenance of regulatory T cells. *Biomaterials, 59*, 172–181. https://doi.org/10.1016/j.biomaterials.2015.04.003

102. Mix, E., Ibrahim, S., Pahnke, J., Koczan, D., Sina, C., Böttcher, T., Thiesen, H.-J., & Rolfs, A. (2004). Gene-expression profiling of the early stages of MOG-induced EAE proves EAE-resistance as an active process. *Journal of Neuroimmunology, 151*(1), 158–170. https://doi.org/10.1016/j.jneuroim.2004.03.007

103. Moore, C. L., Savenka, A. V., & Basnakian, A. G. (2021). TUNEL Assay: A Powerful Tool for Kidney Injury Evaluation. *International Journal of Molecular Sciences, 22*(1), Article 1. https://doi.org/10.3390/ijms22010412

104. Murillo, M., Bel, J., Pérez, J., Corripio, R., Carreras, G., Herrero, X., Mengibar, J.-M., Rodriguez-Arjona, D., Ravens-Sieberer, U., Raat, H., & Rajmil, L. (2017). Health-related quality of life (HRQOL) and its associated factors in children with Type 1 Diabetes Mellitus (T1DM). *BMC Pediatrics, 17*(1), 16. https://doi.org/10.1186/s12887-017-0788-x

105. Muzaffer, U., Ali, S. I., Paul, V. I., & Sheikh, W. M. (2022). Chapter 2 - Immunogenetics: The developmental course. In M. U. Rehman, A. Arafah, Md. N. Ali, & S. Ali (Eds.), *A Molecular Approach to Immunogenetics* (pp. 21–40). Academic Press. https://doi.org/10.1016/B978-0-323-90053-9.00002-6

106. Nami, S., Aghebati-Maleki, A., Morovati, H., & Aghebati-Maleki, L. (2019). Current antifungal drugs and immunotherapeutic approaches as promising strategies to treatment of fungal diseases. *Biomedicine & Pharmacotherapy, 110*, 857–868. https://doi.org/10.1016/j.biopha.2018.12.009

107. Navarro, E., Serrano-Heras, G., Castaño, M. J., & Solera, J. (2015). Real-time PCR detection chemistry. *Clinica Chimica Acta, 439*, 231–250. https://doi.org/10.1016/j.cca.2014.10.017

108. Nelson, W. C., Pyo, C.-W., Vogan, D., Wang, R., Pyon, Y.-S., Hennessey, C., Smith, A., Pereira, S., Ishitani, A., & Geraghty, D. E. (2015). An integrated genotyping approach for HLA and other complex genetic systems. *Human Immunology, 76*(12), 928–938. https://doi.org/10.1016/j.humimm.2015.05.001

109. Nikolajczyk, B. S. (2010). B cells as under-appreciated mediators of non-auto-immune inflammatory disease. *Cytokine, 50*(3), 234–242. https://doi.org/10.1016/j.cyto.2010.02.022

110. Norin, A. J., Mondragon-Escorpizo, M. O., Brar, A., Hochman, D., Sumrani, N., Distant, D. A., & Salifu, M. O. (2013). Poor kidney allograft survival associated with positive B cell – Only flow cytometry cross matches: A ten year single center study. *Human Immunology, 74*(10), 1304–1312. https://doi.org/10.1016/j.humimm.2013.06.027

111. Notarangelo, L. D. (2010). Primary immunodeficiencies. *Journal of Allergy and Clinical Immunology, 125*(2, Supplement 2), S182–S194. https://doi.org/10.1016/j.jaci.2009.07.053

112. Polansky, J. K., Floess, S., Freyer, J., Hamann, A., & Huehn, J. (2009). Epigenetic Regulation of Foxp3 Expression in Regulatory T Cells. In *The Epigenetics of Autoimmune Diseases* (pp. 21–38). John Wiley & Sons, Ltd. https://doi.org/10.1002/9780470743553.ch2

113. Pyeritz, R. E. (2023). Heritable and Polygenic Inflammatory Disorders*. In R. E. Pyeritz, B. R. Korf, & W. W. Grody (Eds.), *Emery and Rimoin's Principles and Practice of Medical Genetics and Genomics (Seventh Edition)* (pp. 321–356). Academic Press. https://doi.org/10.1016/B978-0-12-812534-2.00008-4

114. Rabinovich, G. A., van Kooyk, Y., & Cobb, B. A. (2012). Glycobiology of immune responses. *Annals of the New York Academy of Sciences, 1253*(1), 1–15. https://doi.org/10.1111/j.1749-6632.2012.06492.x

115. Ramos, M. V., Auvynet, C., Poupel, L., Rodero, M., Mejias, M. P., Panek, C. A., Vanzulli, S., Combadiere, C., & Palermo, M. (2012). Chemokine Receptor CCR1 Disruption Limits Renal Damage in a Murine Model of Hemolytic Uremic Syndrome. *The American Journal of Pathology, 180*(3), 1040–1048. https://doi.org/10.1016/j.ajpath.2011.11.011

116. Rashid, T., Mehraj, A., Mushtaq, N., & Rasool, S. (2022). Chapter 1—Origin and history of immunogenetics. In M. U. Rehman, A. Arafah, Md. N. Ali, & S. Ali (Eds.), *A Molecular Approach to Immunogenetics* (pp. 1–19). Academic Press. https://doi.org/10.1016/B978-0-323-90053-9.00015-4

117. Read, S., Hogan, T. V., Zwar, T. D., Gleeson, P. A., & van Driel, I. R. (2007). Prevention of Autoimmune Gastritis in Mice Requires Extra-Thymic T-Cell Deletion and Suppression

by Regulatory T Cells. *Gastroenterology*, *133*(2), 547–558. https://doi.org/10.1053/j.gastro.2007.05.050

118. Redon, R., Ishikawa, S., Fitch, K. R., Feuk, L., Perry, G. H., Andrews, T. D., Fiegler, H., Shapero, M. H., Carson, A. R., Chen, W., Cho, E. K., Dallaire, S., Freeman, J. L., González, J. R., Gratacòs, M., Huang, J., Kalaitzopoulos, D., Komura, D., MacDonald, J. R., ... Hurles, M. E. (2006). Global variation in copy number in the human genome. *Nature*, *444*(7118), 444–454. https://doi.org/10.1038/nature05329
119. Reed, J. C. (2000). Mechanisms of Apoptosis. *The American Journal of Pathology*, *157*(5), 1415–1430. https://doi.org/10.1016/S0002-9440(10)64779-7
120. Reith, W., & Mach, B. (2001). The Bare Lymphocyte Syndrome and the Regulation of MHC Expression. *Annual Review of Immunology*, *19*(Volume 19, 2001), 331–373. https://doi.org/10.1146/annurev.immunol.19.1.331
121. Ribeil, J.-A., Zermati, Y., Vandekerckhove, J., Cathelin, S., Kersual, J., Dussiot, M., Coulon, S., Cruz Moura, I., Zeuner, A., Kirkegaard-Sørensen, T., Varet, B., Solary, E., Garrido, C., & Hermine, O. (2007). Hsp70 regulates erythropoiesis by preventing caspase-3-mediated cleavage of GATA-1. *Nature*, *445*(7123), 102–105. https://doi.org/10.1038/nature05378
122. Robinson, J. H., & Delvig, A. A. (2002). Diversity in MHC class II antigen presentation. *Immunology*, *105*(3), 252–262. https://doi.org/10.1046/j.0019-2805.2001.01358.x
123. Romagnani, S. (2006). Immunological tolerance and autoimmunity. *Internal and Emergency Medicine*, *1*(3), 187–196. https://doi.org/10.1007/BF02934736
124. Rubin, S. A., & Kennedy, R. B. (2020). Paramyxoviruses: Mumps. In R. A. Kaslow, L. R. Stanberry, & A. M. Powers (Eds.), *Viral Infections of Humans: Epidemiology and Control* (pp. 1–57). Springer US. https://doi.org/10.1007/978-1-4939-9544-8_24-2
125. Saito, S., Shiozaki, A., Sasaki, Y., Nakashima, A., Shima, T., & Ito, M. (2007). Regulatory T cells and regulatory natural killer (NK) cells play important roles in feto-maternal tolerance. *Seminars in Immunopathology*, *29*(2), 115–122. https://doi.org/10.1007/s00281-007-0067-2
126. Sakkas, L. I., Bogdanos, D. P., Katsiari, C., & Platsoucas, C. D. (2014). Anti-citrullinated peptides as autoantigens in rheumatoid arthritis—Relevance to treatment. *Autoimmunity Reviews*, *13*(11), 1114–1120. https://doi.org/10.1016/j.autrev.2014.08.012
127. Sant, A. J. (2019). 6 - Overview of T-Cell Recognition: Making Pathogens Visible to the Immune System. In R. R. Rich, T. A. Fleisher, W. T. Shearer, H. W. Schroeder, A. J. Frew, & C. M. Weyand (Eds.), *Clinical Immunology (Fifth Edition)* (pp. 93-106.e1). Elsevier. https://doi.org/10.1016/B978-0-7020-6896-6.00006-5
128. Saravanan, P., & Dayan, C. M. (2001). THYROID AUTOANTIBODIES. *Endocrinology and Metabolism Clinics of North America*, *30*(2), 315–337. https://doi.org/10.1016/S0889-8529(05)70189-4
129. Schneider, S. C., & Sercarz, E. E. (1997). Antigen Processing Differences Among APC. *Human Immunology*, *54*(2), 148–158. https://doi.org/10.1016/S0198-8859(97)00079-7
130. Schreiber, T. H. (2016). Parallel Costimulation of Effector and Regulatory T Cells by OX40, GITR, TNFRSF25, CD27, and CD137: Implications for Cancer Immunotherapy. In P. D. Rennert (Ed.), *Novel Immunotherapeutic Approaches to the Treatment of Cancer: Drug Development and Clinical Application* (pp. 59–78). Springer International Publishing. https://doi.org/10.1007/978-3-319-29827-6_3

131. Serre, G. (2001). From perinuclear factor to citrulline, a target structure for autoantibodies in rheumatoid arthritis. *Arthritis Research & Therapy*, *3*(2), L012. https://doi.org/10.1186/ar159

132. Sinha, S., Itani, F. R., & Karandikar, N. J. (2014). Immune regulation of multiple sclerosis by CD8+ T cells. *Immunologic Research*, *59*(1), 254–265. https://doi.org/10.1007/s12026-014-8529-9

133. Slatko, B. E., Albright, L. M., Tabor, S., & Ju, J. (1999). DNA Sequencing by the Dideoxy Method. *Current Protocols in Molecular Biology*, *47*(1), 7.4A.1-7.4A.39. https://doi.org/10.1002/0471142727.mb0704as47

134. Sonnberger, J., Kasper, L., Lange, T., Brunke, S., & Hube, B. (2024). "We've got to get out"—Strategies of human pathogenic fungi to escape from phagocytes. *Molecular Microbiology*, *121*(3), 341–358. https://doi.org/10.1111/mmi.15149

135. Speth, C., Lass Flörl, C., & Würzner, R. (2007). Complement in fungal infections and complement evasion strategies. In G. D. Brown & M. G. Netea (Eds.), *Immunology of Fungal Infections* (pp. 177–199). Springer Netherlands. https://doi.org/10.1007/1-4020-5492-0_8

136. Steeve, K. T., Marc, P., Sandrine, T., Dominique, H., & Yannick, F. (2004). IL-6, RANKL, TNF-alpha/IL-1: Interrelations in bone resorption pathophysiology. *Cytokine & Growth Factor Reviews*, *15*(1), 49–60. https://doi.org/10.1016/j.cytogfr.2003.10.005

137. Stojanova, J., Pouché, L., & Picard, N. (2016). Genetic polymorphisms in the immune response: A focus on kidney transplantation. *Clinical Biochemistry*, *49*(4), 363–376. https://doi.org/10.1016/j.clinbiochem.2015.07.016

138. Stritesky, G. L., Jameson, S. C., & Hogquist, K. A. (2012). Selection of Self-Reactive T Cells in the Thymus. *Annual Review of Immunology*, *30*(Volume 30, 2012), 95–114. https://doi.org/10.1146/annurev-immunol-020711-075035

139. Suda, T., & Nagata, S. (1997). Why do defects in the Fas-Fas ligand system cause autoimmunity? *Journal of Allergy and Clinical Immunology*, *100*(6, Supplement), S97–S101. https://doi.org/10.1016/S0091-6749(97)70013-7

140. Sun, F., Yang, C.-L., Wang, F.-X., Rong, S.-J., Luo, J.-H., Lu, W.-Y., Yue, T.-T., Wang, C.-Y., & Liu, S.-W. (2023). Pancreatic draining lymph nodes (PLNs) serve as a pathogenic hub contributing to the development of type 1 diabetes. *Cell & Bioscience*, *13*(1), 156. https://doi.org/10.1186/s13578-023-01110-7

141. Sun, T., Jia, M., Wang, L., Li, Z., Lin, Z., Wei, C., Pei, J., & Li, H. (2022). DAR-PCR: A new tool for efficient retrieval of unknown flanking genomic DNA. *AMB Express*, *12*(1), 131. https://doi.org/10.1186/s13568-022-01471-1

142. Süsal, C., & Opelz, G. (2012). Impact of HLA Matching and HLA Antibodies in Organ Transplantation: A Collaborative Transplant Study View. In F. T. Christiansen & B. D. Tait (Eds.), *Immunogenetics: Methods and Applications in Clinical Practice* (pp. 267–277). Humana Press. https://doi.org/10.1007/978-1-61779-842-9_15

143. Teoh, F., & Pavelka, N. (2016). How Chemotherapy Increases the Risk of Systemic Candidiasis in Cancer Patients: Current Paradigm and Future Directions. *Pathogens*, *5*(1), Article 1. https://doi.org/10.3390/pathogens5010006

144. Thomas, D. C. (2017). The phagocyte respiratory burst: Historical perspectives and recent advances. *Immunology Letters*, *192*, 88–96. https://doi.org/10.1016/j.imlet.2017.08.016

145. Torres-Aguilar, H., Blank, M., Jara, L. J., & Shoenfeld, Y. (2010). Tolerogenic dendritic cells in autoimmune diseases: Crucial players in induction and prevention of autoimmunity. *Autoimmunity Reviews, 10*(1), 8–17. https://doi.org/10.1016/j.autrev.2010.07.015

146. Trajanoski, D., & Fidler, S. J. (2012). HLA Typing Using Bead-Based Methods. In F. T. Christiansen & B. D. Tait (Eds.), *Immunogenetics: Methods and Applications in Clinical Practice* (pp. 47–65). Humana Press. https://doi.org/10.1007/978-1-61779-842-9_4

147. Tronik-Le Roux, D., Daouya, M., Jacquier, A., Schenowitz, C., Desgrandchamps, F., Rouas-Freiss, N., & Carosella, E. D. (2022). The HLA-G immune checkpoint: A new immuno-stimulatory role for the α1-domain-deleted isoform. *Cellular and Molecular Life Sciences, 79*(6), 310. https://doi.org/10.1007/s00018-022-04359-2

148. Truedsson, L. (2015). Classical pathway deficiencies – A short analytical review. *Molecular Immunology, 68*(1), 14–19. https://doi.org/10.1016/j.molimm.2015.05.007

149. Tuin, J., Sanders, J.-S. F., Buhl, B. M., van Beek, A. P., & Stegeman, C. A. (2013). Androgen deficiency in male patients diagnosed with ANCA-associated vasculitis: A cause of fatigue and reduced health-related quality of life? *Arthritis Research & Therapy, 15*(5), R117. https://doi.org/10.1186/ar4297

150. Uematsu, S., & Akira, S. (2006). PRRs in pathogen recognition. *Central European Journal of Biology, 1*(3), 299–313. https://doi.org/10.2478/s11535-006-0024-4

151. van der Does, A. M., Hiemstra, P. S., & Mookherjee, N. (2019). Antimicrobial Host Defence Peptides: Immunomodulatory Functions and Translational Prospects. In K. Matsuzaki (Ed.), *Antimicrobial Peptides: Basics for Clinical Application* (pp. 149–171). Springer. https://doi.org/10.1007/978-981-13-3588-4_10

152. von Bubnoff, D., Geiger, E., & Bieber, T. (2001). Antigen-presenting cells in allergy. *Journal of Allergy and Clinical Immunology, 108*(3), 329–339. https://doi.org/10.1067/mai.2001.117457

153. Wellington, M., Koselny, K., Sutterwala, F. S., & Krysan, D. J. (2014). *Candida albicans* Triggers NLRP3-Mediated Pyroptosis in Macrophages. *Eukaryotic Cell, 13*(2), 329–340. https://doi.org/10.1128/ec.00336-13

154. Werfel, T., Allam, J.-P., Biedermann, T., Eyerich, K., Gilles, S., Guttman-Yassky, E., Hoetzenecker, W., Knol, E., Simon, H.-U., Wollenberg, A., Bieber, T., Lauener, R., Schmid-Grendelmeier, P., Traidl-Hoffmann, C., & Akdis, C. A. (2016). Cellular and molecular immunologic mechanisms in patients with atopic dermatitis. *Journal of Allergy and Clinical Immunology, 138*(2), 336–349. https://doi.org/10.1016/j.jaci.2016.06.010

155. Wetzler, L. M., & Guttormsen, H.-K. (2004). B-Lymphocyte Activation and Antibody Production. In *Immunology, Infection, and Immunity* (pp. 233–258). John Wiley & Sons, Ltd. https://doi.org/10.1128/9781555816148.ch10

156. Wiener, A. S. (1966). The Blood Groups. Three Fundamental Problems—Serology, Genetics and Nomenclature. *Blood, 27*(1), 110–125. https://doi.org/10.1182/blood.V27.1.110.110

157. Williams, F., Meenagh, A., Single, R., McNally, M., Kelly, P., Nelson, M. P., Meyer, D., Lancaster, A., Thomson, G., & Middleton, D. (2004). High resolution HLA-DRB1 identification of a caucasian population. *Human Immunology, 65*(1), 66–77. https://doi.org/10.1016/j.humimm.2003.10.004

158. Wintergerst, U., Kuijpers, T. W., Rosenzweig, S. D., Holland, S. M., Abinun, M., Malech, H. L., & Rezaei, N. (2017). Phagocytes Defects. In N. Rezaei, A. Aghamohammadi, & L. D. Notarangelo

(Eds.), *Primary Immunodeficiency Diseases: Definition, Diagnosis, and Management* (pp. 245–294). Springer. https://doi.org/10.1007/978-3-662-52909-6_4

159. Yamamoto, K., & Yamada, R. (2005). Genome-wide single nucleotide polymorphism analyses of rheumatoid arthritis. *Journal of Autoimmunity*, *25*, 12–15. https://doi.org/10.1016/j.jaut.2005.09.004

160. Yang, Z., Kong, B., Mosser, D. M., & Zhang, X. (2011). TLRs, macrophages, and NK cells: Our understandings of their functions in uterus and ovary. *International Immunopharmacology*, *11*(10), 1442–1450. https://doi.org/10.1016/j.intimp.2011.04.024

161. Yin, M., Li, C., Zhang, L., Zhang, L., Lin, J., Jiang, N., Wang, Q., Xu, Q., Zheng, H., Gu, L., Jia, Y., Yu, B., & Zhao, G. (2022). Mechanism of antifungal activity and therapeutic action of β-ionone on *Aspergillus fumigatus* keratitis via suppressing LOX1 and JNK/p38 MAPK activation. *International Immunopharmacology*, *110*, 108992. https://doi.org/10.1016/j.intimp.2022.108992

162. Yuan, X., Li, H., Bai, H., Zhao, X., Zhang, C., Liu, H., Zhang, Y., Zhao, B., Wu, Y., Liu, J., Xiang, Q., Feng, B., Chu, Y., & Huang, Y. (2016). The 11β-hydroxysteroid dehydrogenase type 1 inhibitor protects against the insulin resistance and hepatic steatosis in *db/db* mice. *European Journal of Pharmacology*, *788*, 140–151. https://doi.org/10.1016/j.ejphar.2016.05.034

163. Zerbini, L. F., & Libermann, T. A. (2005). Life and Death in Cancer GADD45 α and γ are Critical Regulators of NF- κB Mediated Escape from Programmed Cell Death. *Cell Cycle*, *4*(1), 18–20. https://doi.org/10.4161/cc.4.1.1363

164. Zinatizadeh, M. R., Schock, B., Chalbatani, G. M., Zarandi, P. K., Jalali, S. A., & Miri, S. R. (2021). The Nuclear Factor Kappa B (NF-kB) signaling in cancer development and immune diseases. *Genes & Diseases*, *8*(3), 287–297. https://doi.org/10.1016/j.gendis.2020.06.005

INDEX

C

D

E

R

S

T